They Want to Kill Us
Here's How and Why

Dr Jack King

Published by EMJ Books

Copyright Jack King April 2024
The right of Jack King to be identified as the author of this work has been asserted in accordance with the Copyright, Designs and Patents Act 1988.

Dedication

For Dottie with all my love and my thanks for your invaluable research, support and friendship

'You matter because you are you, and you matter to the end of your life. We will do all we can not only to help you die peacefully, but also to live until you die.'
Dame Cicely Saunders, British Founder of the Hospice Movement

Contents List
Preface by Dr Cicely Marsden
Introduction: Death by Doctor
Chapter One: Liverpool Care Pathway
Chapter Two: Sustainable Development Goals
Chapter Three: Do not resuscitate
Chapter Four: Demonising the elderly
Chapter Five: Creating misery and fear
Chapter Six: The overpopulation myth
Chapter Seven: The myth that we are all living longer
Chapter Eight: We're all disabled now
Chapter Nine: Euthanasia in Belgium
Chapter Ten: Euthanasia in Canada
Chapter Eleven: Euthanasia in France
Chapter Twelve: Euthanasia in Holland
Chapter Thirteen: Euthanasia in Switzerland
Chapter Fourteen: Euthanasia in the UK
Chapter Fifteen: Euthanasia in the USA
Chapter Sixteen: Euthanasia is not painless, peaceful and dignified
Chapter Seventeen: It's all about the money
Chapter Eighteen: Who will be allowed to kill themselves?
Chapter Nineteen: Who will do the killing?
Chapter Twenty: Palliative care is a human right
Chapter Twenty One: Basic Truths about euthanasia
Chapter Twenty Two: Why euthanasia should be illegal and why you should oppose it
Appendix: The Author

Preface

Euthanasia is being promoted as offering dignity and control and a remedy for loss of autonomy. In reality it is being offered with the implicit thought: 'You are taking up space and money needed for someone else. Go and kill yourself or let us kill you.' In countries all over the world the same lies are told. And all over the world celebrities are recruited to help sell the lie that euthanasia is the only way to provide terminally ill patients with a peaceful exit from life. I wonder how many of those who support the concept of 'assisted dying' realise the vulnerability of socially marginalised populations. Euthanasia has already been used to kill poor people, the physically disabled, the mentally ill and children. How many refugees and drug and alcohol abusers have been killed is rather a mystery since the people doing the killing tend to be a little shy about providing accurate statistics. Indeed, in many areas there are no real statistics because people who have killed themselves (or been killed) are listed in the official statistics according to whatever disease they had last. So, someone with diabetes who is euthanized will have died of diabetes and not of euthanasia. Once death by doctor is legalised, we're all on a very slippery slope. Lord Sumption, of the High Court of England and Wales observed 'the legalisation of assisted suicide would be followed by its progressive normalisation, at any rate among the very old or very ill. In a world where suicide was regarded as just another optional end-of-life choice, the pressures…are likely to become more powerful.' In countries where euthanasia has been legalised, the original criteria have already been broadened.

   Dr Jack King, who has a long and distinguished career in medicine, exposes the many unspoken truths about euthanasia, and his excellent analysis of euthanasia is an invaluable addition to literature which is dominated by the pro-euthanasia lobby. This monograph should be read by everyone with an interest in the subject (and that is all of us) but it should be studied particularly carefully by those who promote euthanasia, doctor assisted suicide or whatever else it may be called.

Dr Cicely Marsden

Introduction
Death by Doctors

Over the years there have been many doctors who have actively promoted euthanasia.

One of the most infamous advocates of this specialised variety of suicide was a pathologist called Dr Murad Jacob Kervorkian who became famous (or should that be infamous) for publicly advocating euthanasia.

Kervorkian's lawyer said that the pathologist was responsible for the deaths of 130 individuals though it is claimed, of course, that the individuals themselves took the final action which resulted in their deaths. Kervorkian apparently attached a device to the patient's body and left them to press a button which released drugs or chemicals which ended their lives. One assumes that if patients needed help in pressing the button then help would be forthcoming.

There was much controversy surrounding Kervorkian, and in 1998, he was arrested and tried for his role in the 'voluntary euthanasia' of a man called Thomas Youk.

Kervorkian was convicted of second degree murder and served eight years of 10-25 year prison sentence. It was later alleged that many of the people he helped to die were lonely and potentially depressed.

Today, around the world, politicians are paying doctors to do what Kervorkian was sent to prison for just a quarter of a century ago. And that is nothing short of obscene. It is absurd that doctors should be involved in euthanasia programmes, whatever they are called. And it is absurd that the favoured term is usually 'Doctor Assisted Death'. The people who enthuse over euthanasia like to avoid the word 'suicide' wherever they can. They seem to think it carries too much unpleasant baggage. Actually, if the words 'euthanasia' and 'suicide' are to be avoided then I prefer the phrase 'Death by Doctor' which is sharp, snappy and entirely accurate.

Attempts are made to differentiate between euthanasia and assisted suicide. The European Association for Palliative Care defines the former as a process by which a medical professional actively ends a patient's life by some medical means in response to a patient's voluntary and competent request, whereas assisted suicide refers to a person intentionally helping another person to terminate his or her life at that person's voluntary and competent request. The differences are legal rather than practical, and various other terms are used in different parts of the world. In New Zealand the term 'assisted dying' is used to cover everything and although that is an honest and straightforward phrase, I still prefer the more honest 'death by doctor'.

It has been said that social engineering is always preceded by verbal engineering, and nowhere is this truism more accurate than in the realm of death by doctor.

Pollsters investigating euthanasia on behalf of lobbyists promoting this form of death use clever phrases to produce evidence that people want more euthanasia. So, they tend to refer to 'death by dignity' because this phrase produces more positive responses than anything containing the word 'suicide'. Phrases containing the words 'compassion', 'freedom' and 'peace' work well and are universally popular.

When professionals want to hide the truth from the public they always invent jargon or terminology. The one word to be aware of this day is 'driver'. When doctors and nurses talk about drivers these days they aren't referring to racing cars or men in peaked hats – they're talking about a device designed to deliver a drug via a syringe. When you hear a doctor or nurse talk about a 'syringe driver' or a 'driver' in the presence of an elderly or sick patient, think about death – it isn't far away.

My big worry is that allowing, encouraging or forcing doctors to become involved in euthanasia creates huge conflicts of interests.

The most important principle of medical practice is 'First, do no harm'. That comes from Hippocrates, now largely forgotten and certainly ignored, but still the Father of Medicine for many and the creator of the original medical code.

By pushing doctors into killing their patients, the legislators and the lobbyists have put doctors into an impossible position. The freedom for anyone to kill themselves has become a right.

The doctor's responsibility is to provide his patient with the best possible diagnosis and treatment. His job is to help his patient. But under euthanasia laws the doctor is expected to offer to help his patient die. And he must then make a judgement about what is best for the patient: life or death. Finally, having been the advocate for life and the advocate for death and the judge, the doctor is expected to be the executioner. This is killing not caring.

Most doctors (and all good, honest ones) reject this new role. In America, the major medical associations and organisations oppose the very idea of 'death by doctor'.

But.

And the BUT should be printed six inches high in red ink.

But you only need a few dozen doctors to agree that killing patients is a good thing to do in order to sustain a euthanasia programme. A few dozen doctors working full time could easily kill thousands of patients. And it is naïve not to assume that the position of legal assassin will attract a good number of doctors who viewed Dr Shipman's career with envy. The medical profession is not free of psychopaths and it is naïve to assume that it is or ever could be.

Moreover, medical schools are now teaching students how to kill their patients. Doctors and nurses are taught to give their patients a catalogue of all the things that can go wrong if they undergo treatment. The same trick is used to 'sell' DNR notices.

And nurses too are being recruited as State assassins.

Partly because of the problem of finding enough doctors prepared to spend their lives killing their patients, the legislation around the world usually includes the phrase 'nurse practitioner' alongside 'medical practitioner'.

This means that a nurse will be allowed to decide that a patient should die, and will then administer the kill shot.

Just what this will do to the image of nursing as a caring profession is difficult to estimate. It seems pretty clear, however, that hospital patients and patients at home are going to view nurses rather differently when they realise that the nurse who approaches their bed with a syringe and needle at the ready may be about to administer the coup de grace.

Those who believe that nurses would not allow themselves to be involved in the murder of their patients (with or without their comprehending permission) should remember that during the unnecessary and damaging lockdowns which were introduced during the pandemic of 2020, nurses and care home assistants gave tens of thousands of lethal kill shots to patients – and then officially put their deaths down as being caused by covid.

Around the world, hundreds of thousands of patients were killed this way without ever having the opportunity to decide whether or not they wanted to be killed.

Those deaths were not suicide – they were murder by nurse.

And it's important to remember that, as with doctors, not all nurses need to abandon their responsibilities for assisted suicide to succeed. And to remember that the nurses who enrol as assassins will be well rewarded financially for their efforts. In health care these days you must never forget the money. It's always there, looming and menacing and influential.

Remember too that for years now, nurses (and care home staff) have been legally allowed to give dangerous sedatives and tranquillisers to people they are employed to look after.

Most worrying of all, perhaps, is the fact that in Canada, doctors who are conscientious objectors (in that they refuse to take part in the euthanasia programme) are obliged by law to refer patients to doctors who are prepared to kill them. If doctors do not do this they lose their licence to practice. And where two doctors are required to sign a 'death by doctor' form, the enthusiastic doctor will merely ask around until he finds a second doctor prepared to do the deed.

How did we come to this? How has it happened so quickly and with such little real thought?

There are many explanations.

One answer, of course, is that movies and games have desensitised millions to death. And the constant playing of news reports of death and destruction also make death seem normal and even insignificant. The desensitisation has had as damaging effect on young doctors and nurses as any other members of the community and so, sadly, many young doctors and nurses are heartless, unthinking and cruel and see absolutely nothing wrong in killing people. If that is what the State wants them to do then they will do it. And is there an extra fee for signing the forms?

The promoters of euthanasia will often claim that only by killing people can we protect them from dying in intolerable pain. This is a lie which has become widely accepted as the truth. I worked as a doctor in hospital and in general practice. I do not remember ever seeing or hearing a patient die screaming in intolerable pain.

Although the problem of addiction to the opioid painkillers is a recognised problem (thanks largely to the overprescribing habits of a small number of crooked doctors) no doctor working in palliative care would allow a patient to scream with pain. It is a well acknowledged fact that patients do not usually become addicted if they are taking a painkiller for genuine physical pain rather than for a temporary 'high'. Moreover, it doesn't matter a damn if a dying patient becomes addicted to a drug. Today it is usual to give patients who are in pain, control of their own medication. By pressing a button the patient can release another dose of their painkiller. There is no longer any need for any patient to scream in pain. (If, however, a dying patient is screaming in pain then it's simply because their pain is being poorly managed, and, sadly, this will happen more and more in a deliberate attempt to steer patients into opting for euthanasia).

Even where euthanasia is not yet legal (as in the UK, for example) people are already being harassed to allow medical and nursing staff to put Do Not Resuscitate (DNR) notices onto their medical notes. This is the first stage towards euthanasia, and there is a terrifying amount of evidence showing that health professionals in both primary care and hospital care have put massive pressure on patients to accept DNR notices. In order to persuade patients to accept DNR notices, doctors and nurses regularly lie to patients ('If you need resuscitation it will be very painful. It's much better for you if we don't attempt to save your life.')

I have absolutely no doubt that 'medically assisted dying' will be promoted in the same way. Encouraging patients to kill themselves is much easier than having to bother diagnosing and treating them.

If you feel that I am being unkind to the once revered healing professions let me remind you, yet again, that during the covid lockdowns, huge numbers of patients were routinely murdered with 'kill shots' consisting of an opioid and a benzodiazepine. (Morphine and midazolam were the favourite tools of death.)

And the patients who were killed were murdered without being told what was happening.

DNR notices may be all that there are in some parts of the world but in numerous countries around the world, euthanasia programmes have been introduced in order to eliminate the elderly and the sick by encouraging them to end their lives. (Life, it seems, is imitating art, for in 1953, Evelyn Waugh wrote a novel called Love Among the Ruins in which he described a state-run euthanasia centre.)

In Trudeau's Canada, the Government has introduced a very forceful euthanasia programme called 'medical assistance in dying'. There were 13,000 state sanctioned 'suicides' in Canada in 2022, and that country is now deciding whether to allow children and the mentally ill to kill themselves. Please read that sentence again. You may need to lie down when you realise the importance of those words. Check it out online if you don't believe me.

In Canada, where euthanasia was introduced several years ago, killing people is proving very popular with doctors, bureaucrats and politicians. A woman in Canada was reportedly offered a place on her nation's euthanasia programme because of the delay involved in having a stair lift fitted in her home. It was also reported that a Canadian man who was facing eviction from social housing had been accepted onto the country's euthanasia program. CBC reported that medically assisted deaths could save millions in health care spending, and it was estimated that the savings 'exceedingly outweigh the estimated $1.5 million to $14.8 million in direct costs associated with implementing medically assisted dying'. The report judged that doctor-assisted death could reduce annual health care spending across Canada by between $34.7 million and $136.8 million. (Just how can anyone take a report seriously when the figures are so vague?)

Today, euthanasia is legal in Belgium, Canada, Luxembourg, Netherlands, New Zealand, Spain, Colombia and parts of Australia as well as Switzerland and some States in America and, by the time you read this, somewhere else as well. Globally, there is a state sanctioned epidemic of euthanasia as governments follow instructions from the conspirators and encourage more and more people to commit suicide.

No one seems to care that suicide is contagious. Once people start killing themselves the idea spreads. Just look at how often one suicide in a school will trigger many more suicides.

And in the countries where doctor assisted suicide (or death by doctor) is legal and commonplace, the number of assisted suicide deaths will be hidden as happened during the false, manufactured covid scare. During the most obscene days of the covid pandemic, patients were officially listed as covid deaths even when they obviously were not. Anyone who failed a PCR test (now recognised as probably the most entirely useless medical test in history) were classified as having covid (even if they had no symptoms of the flu) and if they subsequently died (even months later) they were put down as having died of covid. Abandoning post mortem examinations (for no good reason) meant that it was very easy to list almost all deaths as being due to covid. Patients who were run over by a bus or who died with an axe embedded in their skulls were listed as 'covid deaths'.

Similarly, it is now clear that in countries where official, state sponsored suicide is legal, the number of patients recorded as having killed themselves will be falsified. So, for example, in Canada, patients who have committed suicide (or, more accurately been murdered by a state sponsored assassin) will be listed in the nation's official database by the disease or injury which initiated their progress towards death. So, if a patient with lung cancer ends up killing themselves (or being murdered by the State) they will be officially listed as having died from lung cancer.

And so, just as with covid, no one will really know how many people are involved. With covid the trick was to make the number of people dying look greater than they were.

With euthanasia the aim is to make the number of deaths look smaller and not greater. So deaths resulting from euthanasia are listed according to the patient's previous medical history. This means that a patient who had heart disease and committed suicide will be listed as having died from heart disease. A simple but effective and apparently universal fraud – though just what they'll put on the certificates of people who were euthanized but had nothing wrong with them is something the bureaucrats will have to sort out among themselves. I'm sure they'll manage.

The extreme horrors of euthanasia aren't just found in Canada. In the Netherlands, healthy individuals with autism are allowed the option of euthanasia, and Australia is deciding whether to let children as young as 14 kill themselves (or allow someone to do it for them).

And, of course, in countries which do not yet have legalised, medically assisted suicide, there is always the DNR notice. In hospitals in the United Kingdom, it is now routine for patients who are admitted to hospital to be asked if they want to be resuscitated if they fall seriously ill. Patients are dishonestly warned that resuscitation can be painful and subsequent recovery difficult and that the process may leave them with broken ribs. As a result, many of the patients who are lied to and tricked in this way agree to have 'Do Not Resuscitate' labels put on their hospital charts. Patients who are frail or unable to give consent are often labelled 'Do Not Resuscitate' without the consent of relatives, and the decision not to provide care for patients who are seriously ill may be made by quite junior nurses instead of a team of doctors and nurses as used to be the case a few years ago.

It's difficult to avoid the suspicion that this programme of officially sanctioned mass slaughter is part of a long-time plan to control and to kill – particularly when the stories about doctors doing their best to convince their patients to join the euthanasia movement and making it easier for them to do so.

And it is no coincidence that governments have for years been steadily expanding the definition of 'disabled'. Many of those who have suddenly found themselves able to claim benefits or avoid work may be grateful for the changes that have taken place. What they do not (yet) realise is that the new laws about culling the population are making euthanasia available to everyone who is physically or mentally disabled. Enthusiasm for euthanasia is spreading fast around the world, in just the same way as the unscientific enthusiasm for social distancing, wearing masks, taking a vaccine and so on also spread around the world within hours. Remember, people who've had enough of life can already kill themselves (or, probably more accurately, have the killing done for them) in Holland and Belgium (where euthanasia has been legal since 2002), Luxembourg, Colombia, Canada, Spain, some American states, Switzerland and Victoria in Australia. The list is getting longer all the time.

Who will decide who can or should die? Will it be patients themselves, relatives, doctors, nurses, social workers, teachers, bureaucrats, policemen or just any old neighbourly busy body? Suicide has gone from illegal to optional. When will it become compulsory?

And, remember, there are plans in many countries to allow children (children!) to commit suicide. Naturally, the world being what it is these days, the authorities will not tell the parents of those children what is being planned. The parents will only know after the event, though whether this will be a photocopied letter, a phone call or an email I have no idea. 'You may have noticed that your 12-year-old son did not come home from school today. This is because he enrolled in our Suicide for Students programme and we helped him to kill himself this afternoon.'

How many children (and particularly teenagers) do not sometimes wish they were dead?

'My boyfriend has broken up with me. Now I wish I were dead.'

'I invited Priscilla to the Prom but she's going with Dennis. I wish I were dead.'

'I hate algebra. I know I'm going to fail that exam. I wish I were dead.'

'I've been bullied on Facebook so much. I wish I were dead.'

If medically assisted suicide is made legal worldwide (which I fear it will be) then Pandora's Box will be open. And no one will ever be able to close the lid. It is dangerous to assume that doctors and nurses will also behave responsibly and decently. There is plenty of evidence showing that DNR notices have been put on patients' notes without their permission and even against their wishes. And there is evidence too of health professionals taking advantage of euthanasia laws to kill patients. There is, for example, evidence that one young woman was smothered and suffocated with a pillow – by one or more health professionals.

Mercy killing (as it is also sometimes known) will be like organ donation which started as optional and voluntary but has, in many countries, become the default position, with citizens having to opt out of giving their organs (possibly while they would like to be still using them).

Suicide should not be illegal but just as there is no place for the law in an individual's decision to end their life, so there is no place for medicine. No doctor or nurse should ever be officially involved in any form of euthanasia, and any that does is unfit to remain within the healing profession. There is no place for doctors, the law or the State in suicide. Those who genuinely find living too much of a burden have always been able to kill themselves. Suicide isn't always painless or easy. It is commonly messy and a good deal of trouble. But if the problems of committing suicide are too great then there is a good chance that the would-be suicide will think again. And, who knows, maybe rediscover their zest for living.

Doctors surely kill enough people without encouraging them to do it legally and on purpose. Some decades ago, Dr Vernon Coleman showed that doctors are one of the top three causes of death – up there alongside circulatory disease and cancer. Do we really want doctors to take top position?

Medicine is called 'the healing profession' for a reason. It is not called 'the killing profession'. But wherever euthanasia is legalised, any slender thread of respect which exists between patients and doctors will be severed for ever. And the experiences in Canada show that once 'death by doctor' is introduced, the unscrupulous, the uncaring and the totalitarian will see the system as an excuse to rid the world of people they don't like or don't have any time for. Everywhere that euthanasia is introduced the laws which govern how and when euthanasia is offered are gradually extended. The law invariably begins by limiting euthanasia to elderly, terminally ill patients in severe pain, and before you can blink euthanasia is being offered to people who are deaf or diabetic or 16 and feeling fed up with the world. Patients everywhere now need to be afraid of the softly spoken doctor or nurse who offers them death as a solution.

It is tragic but true that patients are increasingly afraid not of illness or of treatment but of the health professionals who are employed to kill. It isn't difficult to find online film of individuals who have been threatened and harassed and bullied by doctors and nurses trying to 'sell' euthanasia, doctor assisted suicide or, as I prefer to call it, death by doctor. One woman I saw interviewed took her disabled daughter into hospital for help and was offered assisted suicide for her life-loving daughter. When the mother rejected the offer, the doctor told her that she was selfish. Neither the mother nor the daughter had ever asked for her to be killed. 'Do you know how sick you are?' the doctor asked the young girl. (This is a fairly standard question asked by doctors trying to 'sell' euthanasia.) The mother took her daughter home and looked after her with the aid of neighbours within her community.

The criteria for euthanasia are constantly being extended and in some countries children who do not have any fatal disorder will be accepted for death by doctor. Individuals who are merely weary or tired of life are being offered euthanasia, and lobby groups are constantly pushing hard to extend the availability of euthanasia.

There is a general assumption among campaigners for euthanasia that everything done will be done with respect and dignity and that all the health professionals involved will be good people. Sadly none of that is true. Too much power brings out the worst in people and we will be legalising a small force of would-be Dr Shipmans. And the notion that euthanasia (or whatever name is used to try to disguise what is happening) can be guaranteed to be peaceful and painless is a lie. No responsible doctor will claim that euthanasia can or will be dignified or painless. Things can, and do, go wrong with alarming frequency. As one doctor pointed out 'the most dignified and pain-free way to kill patients is to shoot them, but that doesn't seem to be a popular option'.

Many of the people involved in organising 'kill' parties around the world claim to be ethicists. I find this quite extraordinary. How can anyone described as an ethicist promote death by doctor?

Ethics is very simple. You just do the right thing. If you don't immediately recognise the 'right thing', if you don't know what is right and what is wrong, then you cannot possibly be an ethical anything. Those doctors who are killing patients seem unaware that the Hippocratic Oath specifically forbids doctors to administer a poison even when asked to do so.

Can encouraging people to kill themselves ever be ethical, ever be the right thing to do?

It's possible to argue that allowing a patient to die is, very occasionally, the right thing to do. It's even possible to argue that, in extremis, in those last moments, an extra dose of medicine, administered by a caring doctor, can be justified.

But euthanasia as it is being promoted is very different. It's not possible to justify a medical murder which is cold blooded and planned. It isn't possible to justify murder that is promoted or forced upon people

There is some stubborn opposition to euthanasia, I am pleased to say.

Most religions regard euthanasia as wrong. For example, the Catholic Church has insisted that euthanasia is intrinsically evil, and that viewpoint seems unlikely to change. (It is perhaps not surprising that organised religions are routinely being suppressed and demonised.) Priests have been told that they should try to change the minds of those who have chosen suicide. They have also been told that they should not be present at the end if a patient chooses suicide. The Catholic Church insists that chronically ill patients, including those in vegetative states, must receive ordinary care such as nutrition and hydration but accepts that extraordinary or disproportionate care can be suspended if it is no longer beneficial or if it is only prolonging a precarious and painful life.

We should also remember that the vast majority of people who, for whatever reason, attempt to commit suicide and fail, later give thanks that they have failed. With 'death by doctor' that possibility is lost. We should remember too that mistaken diagnoses are now commoner than most doctors will admit. How many people will be killed because they have been mistakenly diagnosed as having a fatal disease?

Can doctors bring up the subject of assisted death without influencing their patients? Or offending them? Or frightening them unnecessarily? Is it really a doctor's job to offer to kill their patient? Will doctors who promote euthanasia be influencing their patients? (Many patients still have enormous faith in the man or woman in a white coat. There's a good deal of trust involved though sadly in many cases that trust is misplaced.)

There is a difference between a patient telling their doctor that they need help sleeping and the doctor then prescribing a bottle full of potentially lethal sleeping tablets, and a month or two later professing shock that the patient has died after a genuinely self-administered overdose and, on the other hand, the doctor sticking a needle into a patient's arm and killing them.

Where does killing patients fit into the duty to care for them?

And it is always important to remember that, despite their claims, and the propaganda spread by its promoters, euthanasia or doctor assisted suicide or death by doctor or whatever else it is called isn't guaranteed to be peaceful or painless.

And contrary to what many people think, euthanasia is, as with so many other things these days, all about the money.

So why is euthanasia suddenly becoming incredibly popular? Why are so many countries making it legal?

I realise that I will be called a conspiracy theorist but I suspect that the people who are behind this obscenity are the same people who are behind the global depopulation plan. There is a powerful group of rich people in the world who feel that there are too many people living on earth and that reducing the population is essential for our survival. This has been proved to be nonsense but conspirators don't ever take much interest in science or logic.

The conspirators claim that it is necessary to reduce the size of the global population, and it is clear that governments everywhere are concerned not just by the size of their ageing populations (and their pension obligations) but also by the overall size of their populations.

And so there are global plans to cut the overall world population down from its current figure of eight billion to a much lower number. Within conspiracy circles, the figure of 500 million (just half a billion) is widely quoted as the number of people that the earth can comfortably hold. This implies somehow getting rid of seven and a half billion people. All of this is based on a tower of lies. Planet earth is perfectly capable of providing more than enough food for eight, ten or twelve billion people. And it is difficult to accept that the world is over-crowded. The certainty is that much of the food is in the wrong place at the wrong time (because of faulty logistics) and many people are also encouraged to crowd into huge cities when there would be plenty of room for them if they were allowed or encouraged to live in or around smaller communities.

It seems to me that the conspirators have two fundamental policies: 'End global poverty by killing all the poor people' and 'End disease by killing all the sick.' Their whole cruel philosophy is actually based on a myth. It was Thomas Malthus who, in 1798, first suggested that the world's population was growing too large and that the Earth's resources wouldn't be able to cope. Gloomily, Malthus predicted starvation, misery and war. But the evidence shows that Malthus was wrong. The world population was two billion a century ago and today it is eight billion but the proportion of people living in abject poverty has fallen from 90% to 10%.

And if farmers really couldn't produce enough food then food prices would be considerably higher than they are.

The irony is that if anything, the problem is that the global population is growing too slowly. Population growth has slowed rapidly in the last half a century, and in western countries in particular the percentage of elderly and dependent citizens has risen rapidly. There are, in short, too few working age citizens around. And the result is that governments are introducing those policies such as euthanasia which are ruthlessly designed to kill off the elderly and the sick (in other words the dependent).

And the situation is getting worse.

Governments and local councils are committed to paying pensions that they cannot possibly ever pay. It is still not widely known but, of course, pensions promised to workers are paid not out of the taxes paid by those workers but by the generation currently working. This has never before caused serious problems but today's younger generation seems to have taken exception to the way things work and have developed an antipathy towards the elderly, forgetting that today's middle aged striver is tomorrow's pensioner.

Chapter One
Liverpool Care Pathway

There have been few more disgraceful innovations than the Liverpool Care Pathway (LCP); a killing programme which was introduced in the late 1990s in a hospital in Liverpool, England, and which has been entrenched in medical care ever since. (I wonder how proud the city of Liverpool is to be associated with this killing programme.)

Caring doctors (sadly, it seems, an ever reducing minority) were appalled when this new protocol was first introduced. It was widely seen as little more than a licence to kill. The LCP was, to put it bluntly, the British equivalent of the gas chambers which the Germans had used in the 1940s.

The Liverpool Care Pathway allows doctors and nurses to withhold food, water and essential treatment from patients who are elderly and who are, regarded as an expensive nuisance.

It is hardly surprising, I suppose, that this officially sponsored disdain for the elderly has trickled through into the British courts. Today, if you beat up a 40-year-old to an inch of his life you are rightly likely to go to prison for a good length of time. But if you kill an 80-year-old you will be unlucky if you go to prison for more than a few months. You probably won't go to prison at all. The lives of the elderly do not count for much. Indeed, you could be forgiven for assuming that the killing of the elderly was regarded as a socially responsible thing to do. How much longer before those who kill old folk are given a knighthood and a free flat in Kensington? This is all particularly surprising since most of Britain's judges are not exactly in the bloom of life.

There are clear policies designed to get rid of everyone who reaches the age of 60 or older. Pensions are kept pitifully small. (The UK's State pension is the worst in any developed economy, and those who rely upon it either starve to death or freeze to death.) Energy prices are allowed to soar so that subsidies can be given to wind and solar energy programmes (satisfying the 'green' lobbyists who care nothing about the elderly) while ensuring that the elderly poor die in huge numbers.

And, exactly as planned, tens of thousands of older people die of the cold every winter because they can't afford to eat and to keep warm.

Eventually, after years of protests, a Government review was commissioned to look into how the Liverpool Care Pathway was working.

More than a thousand families gave evidence, and it became clear that the LCP was being widely used to get rid of sick or elderly patients who were regarded as a nuisance, as 'bed blockers' and as not being worth the effort to treat or care for them. Candidates for the LCP didn't have to be terminally ill or in distress. They just had to be old or disabled – and dependent.

Many patients were, it was revealed, being subjected to the LCP because a prognosis of death had been made. None of the clinicians supporting the LCP seemed concerned that the term 'prognosis of death' is entirely meaningless in clinical terms in that a prognosis is a prediction and it is pretty safe to say that the term 'prognosis of death' can be applied to any one of us.

But once a clinician had announced that a patient in a hospital, a nursing home or a care home was going to die they were, to put it simply, murdered in their bed, usually by being given an infusion of a strong opioid (such as morphine) and a sedative (such as a benzodiazepine). At the same time as the lethal cocktail was given, the medical and nursing staff were instructed to stop all other medication and to stop giving food or fluid to the patient. Most of the patients who were subjected to this regime died within 36 hours, usually in great distress and frequently without anyone (the patient or a relative) giving permission or even being asked for permission.

(Back in 1993, the British courts had, bizarrely, redefined food and water as 'treatment' and this was regarded as evidence that doctors could, on a whim or a fancy, stop patients being given food or fluid.)

However, in 2013, in a report entitled 'More Care, Less Pathway', Baroness Neuberger concluded that 'there can be no clinical justification for denying a drink to a dying patient who wants one, unless doing so would cause them distress…to deny a drink to a thirsty patient is distressing and inhumane.'

It was thought that Neuberger's report would mark the end of the LCP.

But it didn't. To put it bluntly, doctors and nurses ignored it completely.

And so today the LCP is still widely used and although it is impossible to know how many people are murdered in this way, it is pretty certain that the number of deaths occurring this way is increasing every year. During the pandemic of 2020, when the authorities claimed without evidence that a new disorder called covid-19 was a threat to us all, the technique was used very aggressively with the result that countless thousands of patients were murdered with a 'kill shot' consisting of morphine and a benzodiazepine called midazolam. The argument was that thousands of hospital beds would be required to treat all the patients suffering from the 'new' disease (which was subsequently shown to be no more deadly than the standard common or garden flu). In the event, the restrictions introduced during the alleged plague meant that hospitals were quieter than ever, and medical and nursing staff spent much of their time sitting around twiddling their thumbs or making TikTok videos. Don't forget, many of these choreographed dance routines would have required hours of rehearsal beforehand, and yet at the same time we were all being told that hospitals the world over were exceptionally busy treating covid-stricken patients.

The medical profession and the legal profession have defended and protected the continued use of LCP without ever producing any evidence to support the practice. Indeed, when families have gone to the Court of Protection to protest about relatives being deliberately killed in this way, the court has refused to intervene and has also restricted reporting details on the identity of the individuals involved, the staff doing the murdering and the responsible institution. There is no accountability and no transparency.

Sam Ahmedzai, Emeritus Professor of Palliative Medicine at Sheffield University, said 'Dehydrating a person to death is distressing, degrading and inhuman. Having helped to see the infamous Liverpool Care Pathway abolished, I can see the spirit of it lives on today in Britain.'

The recommendations made in 'More Care, Less Pathway' were accepted by the Government but they were not, it seems, accepted by the medical or nursing professions (or, indeed, the legal profession).

The slaughter of patients continues apace today. The LCP was rebranded and has continued, largely in secret.

Once a doctor or nurse has announced a prognosis of death (officially announcing that the patient is eventually going to die), the provision of food and fluids is stopped and kill shot drugs are prescribed and given via a syringe driver. The courts protect such activity, apparently arguing that the doctors doing the killing are always right and that any doctors who question the practice must, almost by definition, be wrong. Moreover, all such discussions are done in camera, and relatives are banned from talking about what has happened. Indeed, one doctor who tried to question a decision to kill a patient was reported to the General Medical Council for trying to save the patient's life. The GMC, a woke organisation which always seems to put the concerns of the establishment above the rights of doctors and the needs of patients, is reported to have taken three years to exonerate the doctor concerned.

Chapter Two
Sustainable Development Goals

If the Liverpool Care Pathway allowed doctors and nurses everywhere to kill their patients with impunity, then the Sustainable Development Goals which the United Nations gave to the world seem to have been devised to whitewash the procedure.

The Sustainable Development Goals are a blueprint for a New World Order (aka the Great Reset). The small-print effectively allows doctors and hospitals to discriminate against anyone over the age of 70 on the grounds that people who die when they are over 70 cannot be said to have died 'prematurely' and so will not 'count' when a nation's healthcare is being assessed.

Governments everywhere love this new rule because it gives them 'permission' to get rid of citizens who are of pensionable age and, therefore, regarded by society's accountants as a 'burden'.

The Sustainable Development Goals are just another example of the anti-old people policy which is prevalent today.

Chapter Three
Do not resuscitate

Many decades ago, doctors agreed that it was wrong to resuscitate patients who were in severe pain and who were terminally ill (or 'terminally, terminally ill' as is preferred these days). Before the introduction of the 'Do Not Resuscitate' (DNR) protocol it was common for severely ill patients to be dragged back to life time and time again. Whenever such a patient stopped breathing (and effectively died) a 'crash team' would be mobilised. Doctors would run to the ward with masses of equipment and the patient would be injected, intubated and (literally) shocked back to life. As a young hospital doctor I was accustomed to seeing patients repeatedly dragged back to life from the brink of death. No one really thought of just letting someone die. If and when a patient died we considered that we had failed – however old and ill they were.

That was then.

Today, the DNR protocol has been expanded and my mailbox has, for years been full of stories of patients complaining of being asked to sign 'Do Not Resuscitate Forms or having Do Not Resuscitate forms signed on their behalf. (These are known as DNR forms or DNAR forms – for Do Not Attempt Resuscitation.)

DNR notices are only inches away from euthanasia and could, perhaps, be best described as 'passive euthanasia'. The doctor doesn't actually do anything to kill the patient. But he doesn't do what he could do to stop them dying.

In recent years, GPs all over the world have been contacting their elderly patients, and those with chronic health disorders, and asking them two questions. Even perfectly healthy patients have been approached if they have reached a certain age. (The age at which doctors consider a patient not worth saving varies but is usually around 70.)

'Are you happy for us to put a DNR on your file?'
And

'Are you happy for us to put on your file a note that you won't be admitted to hospital if you become unwell?'

Note the clever wording, designed to elicit a positive response. It's the sort of trickery used by crooked pollsters and insurance salesmen – knowing what answer they want and shading the question in such a way as to ensure that they get it.

One medical practice sent out a letter to a home catering for autistic adults saying that the carers should have plans to prevent their patients being resuscitated if they became critically ill.

Other GPs sent out similar letters to establishments caring for the elderly and the disabled. Blanket decisions were made for care homes and residential homes caring for patients with learning difficulties.

A 51-year-old man with Down's Syndrome was given a DNR because of his disability, and instructions were left that there was to be no attempt to resuscitate him if he had a cardiac arrest or a respiratory arrest. No consent form was signed and there was no agreement with the patient or his relatives. The Medical Director for the relevant part of Britain's National Health Service said that their policy complied fully with national guidelines from professional bodies.

The boss of a large charity said that they believe that DNR orders were frequently being placed on patients with learning disabilities – without the knowledge and agreement of their families.

This was, of course, illegal.

Back in 2015, the High Court in the UK ruled that carers for patients with mental illnesses should be consulted before DNR notices were applied.

But the coronavirus nonsense resulted in a flood of such cases.

A man in his 50s, with sight loss, was issued with a DNR notice giving 'blindness and severe learning disabilities' as the reason.

A man with epilepsy was issued with a DNR notice, and at the end of March this year a GPs' surgery in Wales urged high risk patients to complete a DNR form if they contracted the coronavirus. The letter said, 'you are unlikely to receive hospital admission'.

A woman in Bristol received a phone call from her GP asking if it were OK for her medical records to be updated to say that if she contracted the coronavirus she wouldn't go to hospital or receive any medical treatment.

In the UK, the National Institute for Health and Care Excellence, known as NICE, is the official advisory body to the health care world. And a NICE ruling is utterly crucial.

NICE classified people in nine categories. If you are in category 1 then you are very fit. If you are in category 9 then you are terminally ill (though, when it suits them NHS staff sometimes devise another category of 'terminally, terminally ill').

On 29th April 2020, NICE issued amended advice to NHS staff about its resuscitation guidelines, saying that doctors should 'sensitively discuss a possible DNAR with all adults with CFs of 5 or more'. This was issued in response to the coronavirus hoax. Doctors and nurses were instructed that they should review critical care treatment when a patient 'is no longer considered able to achieve desired overall goals'.

So, what does this mean?

And what is a CF? What does a CF of 5 mean?

Well, the letters CF mean clinical frailty and there are several stages.

A CF of 5 means that a patient is mildly frail and may need help with heavy housework, shopping and preparing meals.

A CF of 6 means moderately frail – people who need help with bathing.

A CF of 7 means severely frail – people who are completely dependent for personal care.

And so on.

Now you could, I suppose, argue that if a patient is clearly dying then it would be cruel and pointless to continually attempt resuscitation. That was why DNR notices were devised. They were originally for patients who had only minutes or possibly hours to live, and it was considered not fair to those patients to continue to 'strive to keep officiously alive'.

But that's not what is happening now.

Today, in the UK, in the National Health Service a patient is officially considered unsuitable to be saved or treated if they need help with heavy housework or if they have difficulty preparing meals or going to the shops.

I could manage a bit of light dusting, I suppose, but more than that would require more effort than I have available to spend on such matters. I would have great difficulty in preparing a meal and I hate going to the shops. So, presumably, I'd get dumped into the CF5 category. And, in that case, there is no hope for me, and the NHS would recommend that I be denied antibiotics, painkillers or surgery if I fell down and broke an arm.

The post-coronavirus hoax NHS doesn't want to save anyone who is disabled, and all patients in care homes are, by definition, suitable for murder by omission.

Originally NICE told doctors that they should assess patients with autism as scoring high for frailty. I am, I confess, still rather confused about when or whether this advice was removed.

I checked around and found that the General Medical Council, which provides doctors with their licences, had got in on the act by defining 'approaching end of life' as patients who are likely to die within the next twelve months.

This, of course is the sort of dangerous rubbish one might expect from the overpaid bureaucratic form shufflers at the General Medical Council because it is always impossible to say that a patient is going to die within twelve months. It may be possible to say that a patient might die within twelve hours but not twelve months. Only very arrogant doctors and ignorant bureaucrats claim to know that a patient might die within twelve months. When I was in general practice, I knew many patients who were given months to live but who lived many, many years. Two, I remember well, had young children to look after and although they had been given only months to live they both lived for years – simply refusing to give up and surviving on sheer willpower as much as anything else. If the GMC rule had been applied, they'd have been allowed to die. Or, the way things seem to be going, they would have been quietly euthanized in case they fell ill and needed care.

While digging around I also found this statement: 'Physicians have been empowered to grant a mercy death to patients considered incurable – the mentally ill and the handicapped.'

And then I looked a little closer and realised that the date of that policy statement was October 1939, and the author was a well-known 'medical expert' known as Adolf Hitler.

Hitler's policy, which seems to me to bear an uncomfortably close relationship to the official policy of the UK's National Health Service these days, was created in 1920 in a book written by a psychiatrist and a lawyer (what a deadly combination) who argued that the economic savings justified killing those with 'useless lives'.

The policy was to kill the incurably ill and the physically or mentally disabled and the elderly.

Hitler's policy was officially discontinued in 1941 when it seems that even the Nazis found it a bit much.

But the advice from NICE is still valid. And the NHS is still prepared to refuse life-saving treatment for the elderly, the disabled or the frail.

Refusing treatment to patients solely because of their age or fitness is a form of eugenics. It seems that social cleansing is alive and well in Britain today. If you aren't saving people (when you could do so) then you are killing them. There doesn't seem to me to be all that much difference between the thinking behind the policy of Britain's health service and the policy of Adolf Hitler's Germany.

If you slap a DNR form on a patient, with or without their permission, you are condemning them to death.

During the covid nonsense, obedient souls around the world, from New York to London, were witlessly clapping nurses and doctors but all the time those same nurses and doctors were deliberately delivering death notices, DNR forms, to the frail and the elderly.

People shouldn't have been clapping – they should have been clicking their heels and snapping off fancy salutes.

Which of us gave doctors permission to behave like Nazis and to deny treatment to people considered unimportant, expensive or expendable?

In my view, every single doctor or nurse or administrator who has put a DNR notice on a patient under these regulations should be fired, arrested and imprisoned.

How do these people sleep at night? Don't they feel anything for the people they are supposed to be looking after? The people who were scattering these DNR notices around were paid to look after people. And they have betrayed those people. Do Not Resuscitate notices were devised to ensure that the genuinely terminally ill were allowed to die with dignity – without being dragged time and time again from wherever they were heading. DNR notices were originally a necessary part of medicine – to avoid General Franco type situations.

But now we have a thousand Dr Mengele clones working in the health service. That sounds as if I'm exaggerating but the sad thing is that I am not. Dr Mengele would have thrived in today's NHS. He'd have liked the clapping and the adulation too.

NICE should be disbanded immediately. We'd all be better off without it.

Meanwhile, if you live in Britain and you think that you could be rated C5 or worse, it might be a good idea to ask your doctor if you've been put on the 'suitable for dying' list.

Chapter Four
Demonising the elderly

Ageism is rife. Elder abuse is now common, with older citizens being bullied and harassed and demonised when they are at their most vulnerable; frail and in need of caring, support, sympathy, patience and understanding.

The elderly and the poor will be demonised and made to feel guilty if they don't submit to euthanasia. Conditioning, propaganda and predictive programming are all being used to promote the idea that older citizens have a duty to die when they reach 70 years of age. Young people (by which I mean both the Z generation and the millennials) are encouraged to loathe anyone over 60 and to blame them for everything they feel is unsatisfactory in their own lives.

Nowhere is ageism more obvious than in health care. In the UK, the elderly have been abandoned. Women having sex change operations on the NHS are now being given free fertility treatment so that they can have babies after they become men. There is plenty of money to pay nursery school fees for rich parents but no money to provide care for the elderly. Britain's health service has the staff, the time and the money to provide free gender ID clinics, but the elderly are not allowed to have cataract operations under the NHS until they are virtually blind (the authorities clearly hope that they will either be dead or too old for surgery). This absurd policy means that old people denied such surgery cannot look after themselves, and need to be cared for – usually by relatives or neighbours since the State won't do that these days. No one in authority cares a damn about the quality of life of septuagenarians who are unable to feed themselves, read, use the internet or watch television. The politicians and the bureaucrats do not have the wit or imagination to realise that one day they too may be unable to feed themselves, use the internet or watch television.

And, of course, very little money is spent on properly diagnosing and preventing dementia. Alzheimer's is the default diagnosis (GPs are paid a fee for every diagnosis of Alzheimer's which they record) even though many other causes of dementia are treatable if diagnosed. And no one cares about the old people who haven't been officially diagnosed as demented, because they aren't yet quite that far gone, but who find daily life wavering between difficult and impossible in our increasingly demanding, aggressive and threatening age.

The Royal College of Emergency Medicine (RCEM) has said that vulnerable, elderly patients are being forced to wait longer than other patients when they need urgent medical help because hospitals are being bribed with bonuses of up to £2 million if they achieve Accident and Emergency targets set by the Government. Dr Adrian Boyle, president of the RCEM, has said that the immediate short term financial rewards are short sighted and unhelpful. The NHS has set a target of 76% of patients attending A&E to be admitted, transferred or discharged within four hours. (The older, official target was 95% but that has been abandoned because it hasn't been hit since 2015.) Dr Boyle said that 'everyone focuses on the quick wins and the easier patients, and we know that far too many people, once they have waited beyond four hours, they get stuck. So we know that last year there were more than 1.5 million people who stayed more than 12 hours in A&E.' The end result is that elderly people are waiting days in pain and agony in A&E departments.

And, of course, ageism isn't just a problem in the UK. It's a worldwide problem, especially in industrialised societies where it is entrenched in all social institutions, particularly those involved in health care systems. The elderly are vulnerable and suffer massively from increased health risks, environmental pressures and economic stresses.

In all areas where assisted dying is legal, most people who are killed are over the age of 65. But they do not die because they are in pain or terminally ill. They die most commonly because of a loss of independence and dignity and because they can no longer enjoy the sports or hobbies which they previously enjoyed. A study in New Zealand showed that healthy older adults who supported assisted dying did so because they were worried about future impairment and dependency and about becoming a burden on others. They also worried that if they lived they might one day suffer intolerable pain. And so they would rather die now than risk an unpleasant future.

Finally, it is also worth pointing out that older people have admitted that their experiences during the covid-19 pandemic had hardened their views on assisted dying. They'd seen (or read about) what had happened to older people during lockdowns and hospital closures.

Despite all this, it is people under 65 who are more likely to support euthanasia. People become less enthusiastic about euthanasia as they get older.

And it has to be said that euthanasia is, for many, an irrelevance. Tiny pensions, too small to live on, and the increasing cost of heating and basic foodstuffs, mean that millions of old people have to choose between eating and heating in the winter months. In the UK, between 60,000 and 100,000 old people die of the cold every winter and those figures are similar elsewhere.

Chapter Five
Deliberately creating misery and fear to make people wish they were dead

The incidence of mental illness is growing faster than ever before. Anxiety over climate change and the Net Zero programme, not to mention the insane ambitions of the conspirators promoting the idea of a Great Reset, have merged with remaining fears and anxieties over wars that could turn into World War III, to create an epidemic of mental illness.

People are being encouraged to fear living more than they fear death.

Worse still, millions of younger people have been encouraged (by celebrities and entitled, self-absorbed members of the British royal family) to regard every moment of temporary unhappiness or disappointment as a sign of a serious mental disorder which must be treated. Doctors in the UK are now writing nearly 500,000 prescriptions for antidepressant drugs to be given to children. (Antidepressants are powerful drugs with many side effects. They are generally considered to be unsuitable for children. And they don't work.)

And many of the medications prescribed and recommended by doctors for the treatment of mental illness are themselves known to be a major cause of mental illness, depression and even suicidal thoughts. For example, anti-depressants such as Prozac are known to trigger suicidal thoughts and have been named as responsible for a number of suicides. The widely prescribed drugs in the benzodiazepine group may also cause far more mental illness than they can possibly cure. Olanzapine, a widely prescribed drug, can cause a feeling of sadness and emptiness and a loss of interest or pleasure in the world.

All the deliberately created anxiety and stress means that it is not surprising that suicide rates which have nothing to do with euthanasia or doctors, are increasing rapidly. Suicide is now the 10th most common cause of death in the United States and is responsible for around 50,000 deaths a year. The suicide rate is highest among men aged 75 years of older.

Suicide is also getting commoner among children and is particularly likely to be a problem when a child has to deal with violence, emotional or physical abuse, family tensions, bereavement, homelessness and so on.

It used to be the case that one in five teenagers suffered from clinical depression at some stage during their teenage years. Today, depression is much, much commoner and is, indeed, endemic. This is largely a result of the fears which have been deliberately and cold-bloodedly created for the purpose.

Apart from created fear, the one other factor which is significant is bullying. Today, much bullying is online and, curiously, those who do the bullying are often as much at risk as those who are bullied. Children and teenagers who are bullied online are three times as likely as their peers to have suicidal thoughts. The bosses of the big social media companies know about this but do nothing about it lest they damage their profitability.

As I mentioned earlier, it is vital to remember that suicide can behave as though it were infectious. When one child commits suicide other children in the same school or the same area may also commit suicide.

The word 'epidemic' is widely used and abused but there is no doubt that there is now a major global epidemic of mental illness and general misery. This is a perfect background for selling euthanasia. And those promoting euthanasia want it to be available for anyone suffering from mental illness.

As laws are extended, and euthanasia (aka mercy killing) is made more widely available, so the number of people who are suffering from nothing more than restlessness, disappointment or a feeling of being 'lost', but who choose to opt for legally approved, medically assisted suicide will soar.

And, remember, the plan is to make euthanasia available to children (without their parents' knowledge or approval).

How many teenagers suffer from moodiness and so on as their hormones churn and they struggle to cope?

How many conveniently placed apps will encourage them to pick up the phone and make an appointment with their friendly local medical assassin?

During recent years we have seen a dramatic rise in the number of people who are consumed by fear. And there is no doubt that the anxiety has been a major factor in the development of mental health problems.

In the UK, an endless series of indefensible and largely pointless doctors' strikes have led to longer and longer waiting lists for tests and treatment – with the result that by the time they are diagnosed, most people who have cancer are beyond effective treatment. Since the UK has had more doctors' strikes than anywhere else, it is perhaps not surprising that cancer survival rates in the UK are poorer than in any other industrialised country.

'It's now too late to do anything about your cancer – but we can offer you an escape through death if you just sign here to apply to be put on our very short waiting list for euthanasia. There's a two year waiting list to see a doctor about your symptoms but don't worry because we can give you an appointment to see a doctor about euthanasia tomorrow morning.'

There is no little irony in the fact that striking doctors are pushing up the levels of misery and despair and thereby preparing millions for eventual death by doctor – all to the delight of the conspiratorial politicians who are desperate to reduce the global population (though themselves, of course, keep having children).

Manipulators have created fear and sadness and a sense of powerlessness and worthlessness. They have created the concept of a life not worth living.

Is it really a coincidence that the subject of euthanasia is being promoted heavily by the media and by politicians at the same time as fear levels are at their highest for a very long time? In the UK, a tabloid newspaper called the 'Daily Mail' has reported that Princess Diana's death has been used in a euthanasia campaign with the slogan 'Diana did not choose her death. In 2024 we should have the choice'

Fear is one of the major causes of mental illness. And mental illness is now being acknowledged to be an acceptable reason for euthanasia.

Chapter Six
The overpopulation myth

Those who use guilt to persuade the uncertain to opt for euthanasia are likely to introduce the idea that the world is overpopulated, and that the elderly, the disabled and the unsuccessful have an obligation to make way for people who can make better use of the world's resources. This quasi eugenic argument can justly be labelled both elitist and racist since the people being asked to give up their lives are usually poor and powerless.

The official argument is that the answer to the overpopulation problem lies with poor countries in Africa and Asia where too many people are gathered, and the myth is sustained and spread by rich Westerners with large families. This makes the accusation of hypocrisy easy to make and difficult to answer. There is, no doubt, a similarity between this argument and the argument that the world is getting hotter and that the only way to solve the problem is for all to use less oil and travel less. Naturally, the very wealthy are allowed to ignore the rules they make and they constantly criss-cross the globe in private jets.

There are many large holes in the argument that the world is overpopulated and that there isn't enough food to go round. So, for example, it is well established that farmers use less than half of the Earth's arable land and yet, despite that, global food production has consistently increased much faster than population growth. Moreover, some of the most populated countries on earth (such as the Netherlands) have nevertheless been traditional exporters of food.

Several food experts have suggested that the earth could easily support a population of 30-40 billion. Colin Clark of Oxford concluded that the earth could supply an American style diet for over 35 billion and that if people ate a Japanese diet, the earth could feed over 100 billion. Roger Revelle, the former director of the Harvard Center for Population studies, estimated that the earth could provide

2,500 calories a day for 40 billion people – even if farmers were using less than a quarter of the available land.

There is now a widely held belief that the problem is not that the earth is too crowded but that there are too few young people around. Many countries (including China and Japan) have recently tried to encourage couples to have more children.

Chapter Seven
The myth that we are all living longer

Those in favour of euthanasia like to claim that doctor assisted suicide is essential because people are living longer and, as a result, the global population of elderly people is growing out of proportion. The only sensible thing to do, the argument goes, is to kill off the excess old people to preserve space and resources for the young.

The easy and often voiced explanation for both the increase in the size of the developed world's elderly population, and the increase in the number of disabled and financially dependent individuals, is that modern medical miracles, produced by the medical profession and the pharmaceutical industry, have produced the change by enabling people to live longer.

The truth, however, is rather different and the medical profession and the drug companies are guilty of a confidence trick of gargantuan proportions.

The fact is that during the last century, doctors and drug companies have become louder, more aggressive, a good deal richer and far more powerful but life expectancy has not changed as a result.

Improved sanitation facilities and better drinking water supplies meant that the number of babies dying – and the number of women dying in childbirth – fell dramatically at the end of the 19th century and the start of the 20th century, but for adults life expectation has not been rising.

In his book 'How to Live Longer' author Vernon Coleman prepared a list of 111 famous individuals – all of whom lived and died before the start of the 20th century. The names were picked at random. Dr Coleman then checked to see how old these individuals were when they died. I've printed the list below (with Dr Coleman's permission) because it shows clearly that life expectation (now between 70 and 75 years in developed countries) has not risen appreciably during the last century. You may find it illuminating to think of any other individuals who died before the start of this century – and to then check up to see how old they were when they died.

Andersen, Hans Christian. Died 1875 aged 70 years.
Aristotle. Died 322 BC aged 62 years.
Attila the Hun. Died 453 BC aged 47 years.
Audubon, John. Died 1851 aged 66 years.
Augustine, St Aurelius. Died 430 aged 76 years.
Bach, JS. Died 1750 aged 65 years.
Beethoven, Ludwig van. Died 1827 aged 57 years.
Bentham, Jeremy. Died 1832 aged 84 years.
Berlioz, Hector. Died 1869 aged 66 years.
Bernini, Gian. Died 1680 aged 82 years.
Bizet, Georges. Died 1875 aged 37 years.
Blackmore RD. Died 1900 aged 75 years.
Blake, William. Died 1827 aged 70 years.
Botticelli, Sandro. Died 1510 aged 66 years.
Brahms, Johannes. Died 1833 aged 63 years.
Browning, Robert. Died 1889 aged 77 years.
Bruckner, Anton. Died 1896 aged 72 years.
Brummell, Beau. Died 1840 aged 61 years.
Brunelleschi, Filippo. Died 1446 aged 69 years.
Canaletto. Died 1768 aged 71 years.
Cardigan, James , 7th Earl of. Died 1868 aged 71 years.
Carroll, Lewis. Died 1898 aged 66 years.
Casanova, Giovanni. Died 1798 aged 73 years.
Catherine the Great. Died 1796 aged 67 years.
Charlemagne, (Charles the Great). Died 814 aged 67 years.
Charles 11. Died 1685 aged 55 years.
Chaucer, Geoffrey. Died 1400 aged 60 years.
Coleridge, Samuel Taylor. Died 1834 aged 62 years.
Confucius. Died 479 BC aged 72 years.
Constable, John. Died in 1837 aged 60 years.
Copernicus, Nicolaus. Died 1543 aged 70 years.
da Vinci, Leonardo. Died 1519 aged 67 years.
Daimler, Gottlieb. Died 1900 aged 66 years.
Darwin, Charles. Died 1882 aged 73 years.
de Cervantes, Miguel. Died 1616 aged 69 years.
de Sade, Marquis. Died 1814 aged 74 years.

Defoe, Daniel. Died 1731 aged 71 years.
Dickens, Charles. Died 1870 aged 58 years.
Disraeli, Benjamin. Died 1881 aged 76 years.
Dostoyevsky, Fyodor. Died 1881 aged 60 years.
Dryden, John. Died 1700 aged 69 years.
Dumas, Alexandre. Died 1870 aged 68 years.
Eliot, George. (Marian Evans) Died 1880 aged 61.
Elizabeth 1. Died in 1603 aged 70 years.
Emerson, Ralph Waldo. Died 1882 aged 79 years.
Engels, Friedrich. Died 1895 aged 75 years.
Epicurus. Died 271 BC aged 70 years.
Euripides. Died in 406 BC aged 78 years.
Francis of Assisi. Died 1226 aged 45 years.
Franklin, Benjamin. Died 1790 aged 84 years.
Galilei, Galileo. Died 1642 aged 78 years.
Garibaldi, Giuseppe. Died 1882 aged 75 years.
George 111. Died 1820 aged 81 years.
Gladstone, William. Died 1898 aged 88 years.
Goethe, Johann Wolfganag von. Died 1832 aged 83 years.
Gounod, Charles. Died 1883 aged 65 years.
Greco, El. Died 1614 aged 73 years.
Grimm, Wilhelm. Died 1859 aged 73 years.
Grimm, Jacob. Died 1863 aged 78 years.
Handel, George. Died 1759 aged 74 years.
Hansard, Luke. Died 1828 aged 76 years.
Haydn, Franz Joseph. Died 1809 aged 77 years.
Henry V111. Died 1547 aged 56 years.
Herod, the Great. Died 4BC aged 70 years.
Hippocrates. Died 377 BC aged 83 years.
Hobbes, Thomas. Died 1679 aged 91 years.
Hogarth, William. Died 1764 aged 67 years.
Humboldt, Alexander Baron von. Died 1859 aged 90 yrs.
Johnson, Samuel. Died 1784 aged 75 years.
Jones, Inigo. Died 1652 aged 79 years.
Kant, Immanuel. Died 1804 aged 80 years.
Khan, Ghengis. Died 1227 aged 65 years.
Khayyam, Omar. Died 1123 aged 73 years.
Kublai Khan. Died 1294 aged 80 years.
Liszt, Franz. Died 1886 aged 75 years.

Longfellow, Henry Wadsworth. Died 1882 aged 75 years.
Macintosh, Charles. Died 1843 aged 77 years.
Marx, Karl. Died 1883 aged 65 years.
Michelangelo. Died 1564 aged 89 years.
Milton, John. Died 1674 aged 66 years.
Montefiore, Sir Moses. Died 1885 aged 101 years.
Monteverdi, Claudio. Died 1643 aged 76 years.
Mozart, Wolfgang Amadeus. Died 1791 aged 35 years.
Nash, John. Died 1835 aged 83 years.
Newton, Isaac. Died 1727 aged 84 years.
Nobel, Alfred. Died 1896 aged 63 years.
Nostradamus. Died 1566 aged 63 years.
Offenbach, Jacques. Died 1880 aged 61 years.
Palladio. Died 1580 aged 72 years.
Pepys, Samuel. Died 1703 aged 70 years.
Plato. Died c.348 BC aged 80 years.
Polo, Marco. Died 1324 aged 70 years.
Rousseau, Jean Jacques. Died 1778 aged 66 years.
Ruskin, John. Died 1900 aged 80 years.
Sandwich, John Montagu, 4th Earl of. Died 1792 aged 74.
Shakespeare, William. Died 1616 aged 52 years.
Sophocles. Died 406 BC aged 90 years.
Stowe, Harriet Beecher. Died 1896 aged 85 years.
Stradivari, Antonio. Died 1737 aged 93 years.
Tennyson, Lord Alfred. Died 1892 aged 83 years.
Thackeray, William Makepeace. Died 1863 aged 52 years.
Titian. Died 1576 aged 99 years.
Turner, Joseph. Died 1851 aged 76 years.
Victor Hugo. Died 1885 aged 83 years.
Voltaire, Francois. Died 1778 aged 84 years.
Washington, George. Died 1799 aged 67 years.
Watt, James. Died 1819 aged 83 years.
Wesley, John. Died 1791 aged 87 years.
Whitman, Walt. Died 1892 aged 73 years.
Wordsworth, William. Died 1850 aged 80 years.
Wren, Christopher. Died 1723 aged 90 years.

There are 111 names on this list. The average age at death was: 72.39 years. And, on average, it is 433 years since each of these individuals died.

The conclusion is simple: life expectation has simply not increased in the last century or so. The biblical promise of three score years and ten has been fairly steady for centuries. There may be more old people around – but that is merely a reflection of the increase in the size of the global population. The key to longevity is getting past childhood.

And neither drug companies nor doctors can claim responsibility for the reduction in infant mortality rates.

It has been the increase in the supply of good food, the increase in the supply of pure water and the improvement in the quality of available housing which has had the greatest effect. A WHO publication entitled 'Life Expectancy in the Year 2000' adds stable government, progress in road building and better education to this list. Cholera one of the biggest 'killers' of the nineteenth century, was brought under control by hygienic measures years before Koch discovered the existence of the cholera vibrio, and the decline in the incidence of tuberculosis was due not to the discovery of the tubercle bacillus but to improved nutritional standards.

Drug companies and doctors may like to claim that they are responsible for the increase in mortality. But the claim is at best disingenuous and at worst fraudulent.

There were over 40,000 deaths from tuberculosis in England and Wales in 1925 but only about 1,500 in 1970. There were over 6,000 deaths from whooping cough in 1925 but only 15 in 1970. More than 5,000 people died from measles in 1925 but by 1970 the annual mortality rate had dropped below 50. The mortality from gastro-intestinal infections has dropped by 80 per cent in the United Kingdom since 1930 and the number of deaths from chest infections has dropped by 70 per cent in the same period. Statistics and charts show that none of these changes was brought about by drugs or vaccines. All were brought about by public health improvements.

The apparent improvement in life expectancy which we have enjoyed in this century has been largely due to the fact that there has been a dramatic decrease in the number of children dying. In 1900, about 150 children in every 1000 born in England and Wales died within one year. By 1950, this figure was down to 30.

Adults, however, have benefited far less from the improvements. If we consider their life expectancy, we find that it has hardly changed in the last three-quarters of a century. The 45-year-old male could expect another 23 years in 1901 and only another 25 years in 1971. The improvement in standards of nutrition and in living standards generally had very much affected the life expectation of the middle-aged man in the second half of the nineteenth century; in the first half of the twentieth century it was the survival rate of infants which was most improved.

Astonishingly, there has been almost no improvement in life expectation for the elderly. A World Health Organisation study has shown, in fact, that in a number of industrial countries, the life expectancy of people over the age of sixty has actually started to fall. In the United States, where expenditure on health care is enormous, life expectancy for men and women of all ages is falling.

The fact that hospital waiting lists are increasing all the time, that the amount of sick leave taken by working men and women seems to rise each year, that mental illnesses are getting commoner, that the incidence of heart disease seems to be on the increase, that there is a massive increase in the amount of pollutant-inspired illness, that 80 per cent of modern cancers are thought to be caused by chemicals of one sort or another, and that the number of health professionals needed to cope with all the sickness is increasing rapidly, seem to suggest that medical research has had relatively little effect on the morbidity rates or upon the quality of life at any time in the last century.

In addition, there is evidence that medical research has actually detracted from the quality of life, causing ethical problems and using funds which could be better used on projects more likely to contribute to good health.

Indeed, there is not only evidence for the uselessness of much medical research: there are also sound indications that many developed countries have reached a point of over-medication which is harmful to health. As Dr Vernon Coleman pointed out in his book 'Coleman's Laws', if a patient has two conditions – two diseases – there is a very good chance that one of those diseases was caused by the treatment for the other.

Writing in the Journal of Human Resources, an American researcher, Charles T. Stewart, has shown that life expectation is approximately the same in countries with between 4 and 16 doctors per 10,000 people. It is a certain fact that while the number of patients treated by doctors is increasing in numerical terms, the number saved as a percentage of those who could be saved is falling dramatically.

There is a savage irony in the fact that we have now reached the point where, on balance, well-meaning doctors in general practice, and highly trained, well-equipped specialists working in hospitals, may do more harm than good. The epidemic of iatrogenic disease which has always scarred medical practice has been steadily getting worse, and today most of us would, most of the time, be better off without a medical profession.

Most developed countries now spend a huge proportion of their Gross National Products on health care but through a mixture of ignorance, incompetence, prejudice, dishonesty, laziness, paternalism and misplaced trust, doctors are killing more people than they are saving, and they are causing more illness and more discomfort than they are alleviating. Most developed countries now spend around 1% of their annual income on prescription drugs, and doctors have more knowledge and greater access to powerful treatments than ever before, but there has probably never been another time in history when doctors have done more harm than they do today.

If doctors really did help people stay alive then you might expect to find that the countries which had most doctors would have the best life expectation figures. But that isn't the case at all.

My view may sound startling and controversial but it is a view shared by a growing number of independent experts around the world. These figures hardly support the image of doctors as an effective healing profession.

Whatever statistics are consulted, whatever evidence is examined, the conclusion has to be the same. Doctors are a hazard rather than an asset to any community. The British were never healthier than they were during the Second World War.

Remove the improvements produced by better living conditions, cleaner water supplies, and the reduction in deaths during or just after childbirth and it becomes clear that doctors, drug companies and hospitals cannot possibly have had any useful effect on life expectancy. Indeed, the figures show that there has been an increase in mortality rates among the middle aged and an increase in the incidence of disabling disorders such as diabetes and arthritis. The incidence of diabetes, for example, is now reported to be doubling every ten years, and the incidence of serious heart disease among young men is increasing rapidly – though this is undoubtedly largely due to the damage done by the covid-19 vaccination programme. The explosion of drugs and surgical treatments for heart disease has had no positive effect on death rates. On the contrary, there is a considerable amount of evidence to show that the increase in the use of such procedures as angiography, drug therapy and heart surgery has resulted in more deaths. People in the West are being doctored and drugged to death.

Four out of five people in the world live in underdeveloped countries but four out of five drugs are taken by people in developed countries. Despite the expenditure of enormous amounts of money on screening programmes, deaths of young women from cancer continue to go up, and every time one infectious disease is conquered, another seems to take its place. Bacteria are becoming increasingly resistant to antibiotics, and the number of disabled and incapable citizens in developed countries is increasing so rapidly that it is now clear that the number of disabled and incapable individuals will soon outnumber the healthy and able bodied.

In Britain, where free access to doctors and hospitals is available to everyone, life expectancy for 40-year-olds is lower than almost anywhere else in the developed world. In America, 6% of hospital patients get a drug resistant, hospital induced infection and an estimated 80,000 patients a year die in this way. This puts hospital infections high among the top ten causes of death in America.

The bottom line is that when doctors and drug companies produce figures which show that there has been a (usually slight) increase in life expectation during the last one hundred years or so, they invariably overlook the massive contribution made by improved living conditions, cleaner drinking water, better sewage disposal facilities, more widespread education, better (and more abundant) food and better and safer methods of transport. All these factors have had a far more dramatic influence on mortality and morbidity rates than the provision of health care services.

Relief organisations working in underdeveloped parts of the world are well aware that they can make an impact on mortality rates far more speedily by providing tools, wells and shelter than by building hospitals or clinics or importing doctors and nurses. Sadly, the governments receiving help are often loathe to accept this simple truth and are frequently much more enthusiastic about building state of the art hospitals complete with scanners, heart transplant teams and intensive care units than they are about building homes, installing irrigation systems or planting crops.

This obsession with high technology leads to problems in all areas of health care. For example, the control of malaria was going well for as long as stagnant pools of water were removed, but when it was discovered that the mosquitoes could be killed by spraying DDT and that the disease could be controlled by using drugs such as chloroquine, the authorities stopped bothering to remove stagnant pools. Today mosquitoes are resistant to DDT, and the parasites which cause malaria are becoming resistant to the drugs. As a result, malaria now kills millions.

From the dark ages, through the Renaissance and up to the first few decades of the 20th century, infant mortality rates were absolutely terrible and it was these massive death rates among the young which brought down the average life expectation. The Foundling Hospital in Dublin admitted 10,272 infants in the years from 1775 to 1796 and of these only 45 survived. In Britain, deaths among babies under twelve-months-old have fallen by more than 85% in the last century. Even among older children the improvement has been dramatic. In 1890, one in four children in Britain died before their tenth birthday. Today, 84 out of every 85 children survive to celebrate their tenth birthday. These improvements have virtually nothing to do with doctors or drug companies but are almost entirely a result of better living conditions. In 1904, one third of all British schoolchildren were undernourished. Poor diets meant that babies and small children were weak and succumbed easily to diseases. Older children from poor families were expected to survive on a diet of bread and dripping, and many women who had to spend long hours working in terrible conditions were unable to breast feed their babies, many of whom then died from drinking infected milk or water.

When the improvements in child mortality figures are taken out of the equation, it is clear that for adults living in developed countries life expectation has certainly not risen in the way that both doctors and drug companies usually suggest.

And, for the record, it isn't possible to credit vaccination programmes with the improvement in life expectation since the figures show quite clearly that mortality rates for all infectious diseases had, as a result of better living conditions, all fallen to a fraction of their former levels long before any of the relevant vaccines were introduced.

Chapter Eight
We're all disabled now

Governments everywhere have been preparing for the Big Cull for some years.

Back in 2010 the British Government changed the legal definition of disability. You may think that like pornography you will recognise disability if you see it. You'd almost certainly be wrong.

You are now automatically classified as disabled (and, therefore, likely to be a suitable candidate for euthanasia) if you have:

Cancer

A HIV infection

Multiple sclerosis

Any visual impairment (even sight impairment or being partially sighted – which would mean that many who simply need spectacles to read or drive might well be officially disabled)

Any progressive condition such as Alzheimer's disease and Parkinson's disease

Any physical or mental impairment which has a substantial and long term adverse effect on your ability to carry out normal day to day activities (the term 'long term' means more than 12 months but long term may also mean fluctuating). It is important to note that children who are physically or mentally impaired may be considered for euthanasia but their parents will not be consulted.

Any difficulty in communicating with other people

Any difficulty in filling in forms

Any difficulty in preparing and eating food

Any difficulty in sitting down or standing up

Any difficulty in using a computer

Any difficulty in writing

Any difficulty in getting washed and dressed

Any difficulty in following instructions

Any disfigurement

Long covid. (Even though experts believe there is no specific disease as 'long covid' and that the millions who are off work complaining of 'long covid' are mostly either skiving or suffering from psychological problems brought about by fear and misinformation. There are a good number of people in society who are vulnerable to developing psychosomatic symptoms. So, for example, if they were told that getting out of bed on a Tuesday would cause all these terrible, debilitating symptoms, and they were repeatedly told this by the media, then very soon they would find themselves bed-ridden every Tuesday. Sadly, this manipulative brain-washing technique is being used more and more with illnesses that were once considered mild, natural or not even illnesses at all).

Menopause (bizarrely many menopausal women welcomed the prospect of allowing themselves to be described as 'disabled' while menopausal women are now legally entitled to insist on working from home, something which may cause problems when the authorities realise that this means that surgeons, nurses, bus drivers, airline staff, shop assistants and professional long distance runners will all be working from home)

Any of the problems now described as examples of neurodiversity (including ADHD, autism, dyslexia, dyspraxia and so on)

Mental illness

All of the people with disorders listed above are candidates for euthanasia, whether they know it or not and whether or not they are willing to be killed. It is worth noting that one in nine children is now officially classified as disabled (and that proportion is rising daily).

Chapter Nine
Euthanasia in Belgium

Death by doctor has been legal in Belgium since the early part of the 21st century with various alterations along the way. One law legalised passive euthanasia (such as withholding artificial life support as a 'right to die') and in another allowed doctors to give patients deep and continuous sedation.

Anything is possible once euthanasia laws have been passed. The courts never find in favour of anyone who objects to what is happening. Once euthanasia begins there are no limits.

Some of those who campaign in favour of death by doctor probably feel they are being led by what they think is compassion.

But most are simply being led by politicians who are leading us all towards the Great Reset. The right to die has superseded the right to live.

Chapter Ten
Euthanasia in Canada

As with the pandemic, the vaccine and the insane, privacy-crushing move towards digital currencies, the move toward euthanasia is global. The two countries which always seem to be at the forefront of developments are Canada and New Zealand. And although it is only now that the enthusiasm for euthanasia and assisted dying seems to be reaching a peak, the ground work has been under way for a long time.

It was in June 2016 that the Medical Assistance in Dying programme became the law in Canada. From then until July 2020, there were more than 13,000 reported medically assisted deaths in Canada. Most alarmingly, nearly 20% of those who were allowed to kill themselves (or who chose to be killed) had received no palliative care support, though it is unknown if any were offered palliative care and refused it.

(The word 'kill', 'manslaughter' and 'murder' never appear in official documentation dealing with euthanasia. It seems to me, however, that avoiding the word 'kill' is simply cosmetic –designed to make everyone concerned feel better about a subject which needs to be dealt with as honestly as possible.)

In March 2021, the Department of Justice in Canada announced changes and introduced a new MAID law which removed the requirement for an individual's natural death to be reasonably foreseeable in order to be eligible for MAID. In other words, Canadians could be legally killed even if they were not terminally ill.

In addition, the new MAID made it legal for persons whose natural death was reasonably foreseeable to fix a set date to be killed and to waive final consent if it was thought possible that they might lose mental capacity before the date that had been fixed for their death.

And a review was then set up to look at making it possible to find a way to help patients suffering solely from mental illness (anxiety and depression and so on) to kill themselves.

Finally, in 2021, the Government of Canada said that it was looking at the eligibility of children for euthanasia.

By the autumn of 2023, the Canadian programme for enabling its citizens to kill themselves was growing incredibly rapidly. The killing of patients jumped 31% in 2022, as the trend accelerated for more and more patients to opt for euthanasia over palliative care. Indeed, the average annual growth for killing yourself was running at 31%.

In 2023, 63% of those who chose to be killed had cancer and 19% had heart conditions, though there does not seem to be any evidence showing how many were close to death or in untreatable pain. The number who had received palliative care was 78% and half of the patients who received palliative care received it for less than a month.

Again nearly 20% of the patients who were killed had received no palliative care at all, so if they had pain they had not received the appropriate help.

Astonishingly, over four per cent of ALL deaths in Canada in 2023 were due to euthanasia. And the Government was by then planning to extend eligibility.

The report also noted that the lack of trained MAID providers has been a concern due to the growth in applicants. Just under 10% of the killing was done by a nurse with no doctor present, suggesting that both the curing and caring professions had abandoned their traditional roles.

In Canada and some other countries, you don't have to have a fatal illness to qualify for the euthanasia programme. You can choose to die just because you've had enough of life. Or because you have been convinced that killing yourself is the decent thing to do

A psychiatrist noted that in 2022, nearly 500 of those who were killed 'did not have reasonably foreseeable deaths' but were killed anyway. The 2022 figure was around twice the number who did not have reasonably foreseeable deaths but were killed in 2021.

I would make two points.

First, it is very rarely possible to decide that a patient's death is foreseeable. Like all doctors I have frequently seen patients make a recovery after being described as 'terminally, terminally' ill and beyond medical help. (The phrase 'terminally, terminally ill' is now being used by bureaucrats with no medical training to describe patients who are considered by them to be close to the end of their lives.)

Second, in some countries (notably the UK) the new laws about 'disability' mean that almost anyone can now be described as having an illness, disease or disability. So, for example, now that menopausal women are defined as being disabled it would be possible to push them into a suicide programme.

One third of those taking part in Canada's euthanasia programme perceived themselves to be a burden on their family, their friends and on caregivers. A number also expressed concern about the amount of money that was being spent on caring for them when they could no longer contribute to society.

There is no doubt that guilt will be used as a weapon to persuade the disabled, the sick and the elderly to accept suicide as the 'decent way out'

Those who promote the idea of 'killing by doctor' invariably argue that the victims of their enthusiasm are elderly, in pain and at the end of their lives. The myth is compounded by the lie that everyone who is killed this way has chosen their end of life and is guaranteed a painless exit. Neither of these claims is true.

A campaign group called 'Dying with Dignity' claims that the killings are 'driven by compassion, an end to suffering and discrimination and desire for personal autonomy'.

But that doesn't seem to be what is happening in practice.

The fact is that the 'killing by doctor' regime has evolved and now bears no resemblance to the original plan. Many of the people who are killed are young and in good physical health. Canada has seen a massive rise in the number of people being deliberately killed by their doctors, and euthanasia is rapidly becoming one of Canada's fastest growing causes of death. Many patients (and their relatives) have reported that they've been badgered to accept MAID.

'Today, it seems that the concept of wanting treatment is coming, to some medical staff, to be seen as absurd – that you actually want treatment and not death,' said an anti-MAID activist. 'You're now being seen as terrible for wanting to be treated. You're costing the system.'

Here are some case histories which might help you decide whether or not you approve of euthanasia:

Christine Gauthier, a former member of the Canadian military who injured her back in a 1989 training accident and who competed for Canada at the 2016 Rio de Janeiro Paralympics, needed a wheelchair ramp in her home. She'd been trying to get the ramp for five years. The caseworker who responded offered her a medical assisted death (the Canadian version of euthanasia is known as MAID) and offered to provide the equipment. The Veterans Minister, Lawrence MacAulay later revealed that at least four other Canadian military veterans had been offered a medically assisted death. He added that a veterans' service agent had been suspended.

Kathrin Mentler, a 37-year-old counselling student went to the Vancouver General Hospital for help with her debilitating feelings of depression and hopelessness. The staff member she saw told that psychiatrists were in short supply. 'Have you considered MAID?' she was asked. The clinician who made this bizarre and inappropriate offer said that overdosing at home could lead to brain damage whereas a state-administered MAID death would be more comfortable. A Vancouver Coastal Health spokesman, Jeremy Deutsch, said that the hospital had followed protocols.

A 61-year-old woman called Donna Duncan suffered from depression after a concussion sustained in a car crash. She was offered, and accepted, death by doctor as an alternative to treatment. Mrs Duncan's daughters, Alicia and Christie later requested an investigation, saying that their mother should not have been offered death because of her mental health troubles. The police investigation concluded with no arrests.

Alan Nichols, a 61-year-old Canadian was killed by a lethal injection in 2019. His health problem was hearing loss. His brother later said that Mr Nichols was 'basically put to death'. No medical personnel contacted his relatives 'out of respect for patient confidentiality'.

An unnamed Canadian Forces veteran suffering from PTSD was told that he could opt for a medically assisted death. Family members said that the veteran felt betrayed and that the offer had derailed his recovery.

Roger Foley suffers from a degenerative brain disorder and was offered euthanasia so often that he began recording hospital staff. In one recording, a hospital ethicist told Foley that his care was costing the hospital 'north of $1,500 a day' and asked if he had 'an interest in assisted dying'.

After 71-year-old Marilynn Leskun was admitted to Abbotsford Regional Hospital after a fall from her wheelchair, her husband stayed with her nearly 24 hours a day. They had been together for 50 years. He reported later that the medical staff 'pressured' and 'badgered' him to allow his wife to die and then suggested that he let her be euthanized. Mr Leskun said that over an eight day period, staff asked him five times to let them place a DNR designation on his wife. He objected strongly and a doctor then asked him to let staff euthanize his wife. The doctor said: 'You know, I have written orders for medically assisted dying.' Mr Leskun said 'No'. Eventually, worn out by what was happening, Mr Leskun finally said that he would agree to a DNR notice. The nurse replied: 'Oh, it's OK. The doctor has already put a DNR on.' The doctor had put the DNR notice on against Mr Leskun's wishes. Mrs Leskun died shortly afterwards. Mr Leskun said that he believed that MAID is offered 'when the system figures that there is too much cost and effort. I believe that the system has a motivation towards moving those kinds of people towards medically assisted dying.' He went on to say that it seemed to him that MAID was being promoted as a noble choice – 'good for society, for everybody, for yourself, it's the noblest thing you could do.'

Sheila Elson took her daughter to a hospital emergency room in Newfoundland. Unprompted, the doctor informed Mrs Elson that her 25-year-old daughter, who has cerebral palsy and spinal bifida, was a good candidate for euthanasia. When the offer was rejected, the doctor told her that not taking up the State's kind offer to kill her daughter would be selfish.

Lisa Pauli had been anorexic for most of her life. Her psychiatrist assured her that when the laws in Canada are extended she will probably be eligible to be killed by a doctor – because she has an eating disorder.

A woman called Sophia who was living on disability payments and who had failed to obtain affordable housing ended her life under Canada's assisted-suicide laws. 'The Government sees me as expendable trash, a complainer, useless and a pain in the ass,' she said after she and friends had pleaded without success for better living conditions. A second woman called Denise has also applied to end her life because she is struggling to survive on disability payments and cannot find suitable housing. Both women were unable to work and were receiving $1,169 per month – well below the poverty line. When Canada's 'death by doctor scheme' was introduced in 2016, fears were raised that vulnerable groups could be targeted. (I find it scarcely believable but the criteria for MAID were revised after the country's Supreme Court ruled that the previous law which excluded people with disabilities from the death by doctor scheme was unconstitutional. You can always rely on the lawyers and the judges to do the wrong thing, can't you?)

I could go on. But you get the picture. Armed forces veterans and prisoners are not infrequently offered euthanasia.

The really alarming thing is that 73% of Canadians approve of the way 'death by doctor' is being managed. Just 16% of Canadians oppose it. The other 11% have no view and presumably don't think the topic is worthy of their attention.

Just as worrying is the fact that 27% of Canadians believe that MAID should be expanded to include people who aren't ill but who are poor. And 28% of Canadians would offer 'death by doctor' to the homeless. Just 20% would offer MAID to anyone for any reason. Over half of Canadians said that people who couldn't receive the treatment they needed (for financial or other reasons) should be offered 'death by doctor'.

In theory, MAID is supposed to be offered only to people whose problems are incurable. But who knows what is incurable and what isn't? A cure may be just around the corner. The patient's problem may disappear without treatment (as many health problems do). The diagnosis might be wrong (as diagnoses often are). The doctor may not be aware that a cure is available. An available cure may be deemed too expensive.

And with mental health problems, the worries are even greater. We all feel fed up, miserable and down in the dumps from time to time. And when we are at a low ebb, we feel that we will never get better. But something happens, and we feel better. If the doctors in Canada have their say there won't be a chance for a better day. The sensitive and the vulnerable will all be dead.

And 'death by doctor' is to be offered to children. How many children say 'I wish I were dead' without really, really meaning it?

How many teenagers go through glum, sad and sulky periods because of an exam or a failed romance? Are we going to kill them all? Well, it seems that the Canadians are.

The 'death by doctor' regime which is so popular in Canada is promoted not by a far right government but by a notorious left wing government. The result is that the costly, the inconvenient, the unsightly and the vulnerable must all be eradicated.

And think about this: in Canada, the Government has built in provision for instances where patients do not have the mental capacity to decide that they want to commit suicide.

Here's the official wording:

'The medical practitioner or nurse practitioner may administer a substance to a person to cause their death without…immediately before ensuring the person gives express consent…if before the person loses the capacity to consent…they entered into an arrangement in writing.'

If they later change their mind, it's hard luck. They can be legally killed.

Chapter Eleven
Euthanasia in France

Emmanuel Macron, the diminutive (in every sense) French President, has been accused of trying to get rid of sick people by introducing a new law to allow terminally ill people to end their lives in their own homes by taking lethal medication.

'With this bill we are facing up to death,' said M. Macron in March 2024.

Patients who want to enter the killing process will have to apply, repeat their application after 48 hours and then wait up to two weeks for approval from a 'medical team'. Once the approval has been granted, a doctor will deliver a deadly prescription which will be valid for up to three months. Individuals will be able to receive the death drug if they are at home or in any health care facility. If they are not well enough to take the medication they will be allowed to select someone to help them.

This seems to ignore the fact that relatives may find it difficult, not to say traumatic, to give a lethal medicine to a loved one. Macron has said that if the medical professionals rejected the patient's application he or she would be able to appeal or to keep applying to other medical teams (presumably, until they obtained the answer they wanted).

Palliative care workers and nurses said that they were dismayed and saddened by the announcement.

Macron is 'proposing to do away with the sick and to do away with the problem at the lowest possible cost,' they complained, adding that the French President's announcement 'runs counter to the values of care and non-abandonment that underpin our French model of support at the end of life.'

It was also noted that the proposal would doubtless lead to the closure of hospices with many palliative care specialists being made redundant.

The Catholic Church also expressed its discontent. 'Such a law will steer our entire healthcare system towards death as a solution, said Eric de Moulins-Beaufort, the president of the French Bishops' Conference.

Until this law was passed French patients tended to travel to Belgium.

Chapter Twelve
Euthanasia in Holland

Holland is now one of the most dangerous places in the world to be sad, disabled or old.

Dutch doctors have been killing their patients for half a century and it has now become almost normal.

Doctors first put their toes onto the top edge of the slippery slope back in the 1970s but what started as a way to help elderly patients who were terminally ill and in terrible pain has become something much more alarming.

The advocates of killing-by-doctor in Holland don't like to use the word 'kill', of course. Indeed, they never use it. And the word 'murder' would startle them. They much prefer anodyne phrases such as 'physician assisted suicide' or 'aid in dying'. You can call it 'medically assisted suicide', 'doctor assisted death' or 'death with dignity'. Or 'Physician Aid in Dying'. But don't call it killing or murder because the Dutch will be upset. They've mastered the art of state approved slaughter and they're chuffed to bits with themselves.

And there does not seem to be a limit. Doctors will kill people of any age and they will kill people who are demented or depressed. They will kill people who have long-term, chronic disorders. A respected medical journal in Holland has reported that an 18-year-old with psychiatric problems has been killed by doctors.

They will, indeed, kill just about anyone. They'll even kill you if you are just 'tired of life' or 'weary of it all'. A petition, signed by a number of prominent Dutch citizens, has suggested that euthanasia should be available to everyone over the age of 70 who feels a bit worn out and under the weather. Doctors merrily talk patients into being killed for all sorts of reasons. Holland is not a place to go into hospital with pneumonia or a broken arm. Not if you're over 70. Your chances of getting out alive are pretty slim.

Things really started moving fast down that slippery slope when, in 2016, the Dutch Health Minister announced plans for a law that would allow 'assisted suicide' if a patient 'felt that they had completed their life' (whatever that means).

It was said that the needs of older people should be met if they were struggling with mobility problems, a loss of independence, fatigue or loneliness. Meeting their needs shouldn't involve walking sticks, wheelchairs, dietary help or companionship but death by doctor.

The Dutch talk about 'freedom' and 'dignity' but I think they've forgotten what those words mean.

Way back in the 1990s, a 50-year-old social worker felt so miserable that she said she wanted to die. So her doctor gave her a glass of poison to drink. And she duly died.

Back at the top of the slope, patients had to be terminally ill (whatever that means) to be considered suitable candidates for death. There had to be some sort of physical illness. Today, they'll kill you if you are demented or have an existential problem you can't cope with. They'll kill you if you are lonely or depressed or not much good to society. 'Don't worry. Leave it to us. We'll give you something to help you sleep.'

Older patients are made to feel uncomfortable. They're deprived of food, water, diagnosis or medication. And then, when they feel pretty damned uncomfortable and miserable, they're offered a death pill.

'You've had a long life, why are you hanging on when your time is up? You're using up valuable resources. It's time for you to die. They shoot horses don't they?'

The socially vulnerable, the frail, the patients with mental illness are killed because they're a nuisance. You don't have to have a terminal illness or be in pain or be at the end of your tether for them to kill you in Holland.

Iatrogenesis, doctor-induced death, has been one of the top three causes of death for some decades now. The deaths used to be accidental; resulting from a doctor giving the wrong drug or giving too much of a drug. Now the killing is cold-blooded and deliberate.

And they are killing children as young as 12-years-old.

The parents of a child who is contemplating death can be involved in the discussion but their permission isn't required. In Holland it is thought that it wouldn't be right to allow parents to intervene if a child wants to end their life. Children are put down as readily as pets are killed when they are in great pain and cannot be treated.

But there are limits to the brutality. Once the child has been killed the parents will be informed.

Patients in Holland no longer have a right to life.

But thanks to the pro-euthanasia movement, they do have a right to death.

In Holland, the enthusiasts promoting 'death by doctor' now even have a 'Euthanasia Week' where they can share propaganda promoting euthanasia.

The Dutch seem to have taken to euthanasia in the same way that they were enthusiastic about selling marijuana in cafes or sex in shop windows. Anyone over the age of 12 is eligible and there is even talk of babies being accepted for instant death.

Individuals can make a 'Living Will' or 'Advance Directive' in which they sign up for euthanasia at some future time. Anyone who tries to change their mind will, I'm afraid, discover that living wills are legal documents which cannot be easily rescinded.

And the courts are very much in favour of euthanasia. One patient fought back while doctors were giving her a kill shot. The relatives held the patient down while the needle went in. The patient was screaming as well as fighting. Courts later cleared the doctors (and presumably the family) of any crime.

Chapter Thirteen
Euthanasia in Switzerland

Switzerland used to be famous for skiing, banks, cuckoo clocks and chocolate. It is now the place to go to if you want to kill yourself, though, of course, they don't call it killing yourself they call it 'assisted suicide' and there are a number of assisted suicide organisations there to make it as easy as possible.

Despite all the publicity Switzerland gets as the place to go to die, the numbers involved are relatively small with around 1,500 people (Swiss and foreign) choosing to end their lives there.

The comparative popularity of Switzerland as a place to end it all may have something to do with the fact that there were in 2022 just 393 beds available for palliative care in the whole country. This is woeful. The European Association for Palliative Care recommends that there need to be 100 specialised palliative care beds for every one million inhabitants in a country. So, with a population of around 9 million, Switzerland needs more than twice as many palliative care beds as it has.

It's difficult to avoid the thought that if Switzerland provided better care for dying patients it might not have the unenviable reputation as being the easiest place in the world to kill yourself.

Chapter Fourteen
Euthanasia in the UK

Suicide used to be illegal in most countries. Anyone who committed suicide could be prosecuted and imprisoned though it was usually only the ones who failed who were prosecuted since even lawyers and judges realised that there wasn't much mileage to be obtained from prosecuting someone in a coffin. However, the families of those who died could be prosecuted. Suicide was regarded as self-murder and considered a disregard for the will and authority of God. The Church, in its various manifestations regarded suicide as a sin.

Now, of course, suicide is mostly legal and it is becoming increasingly fashionable.

It was only in 1961 that suicide became legal in England and Wales. The law was changed to decriminalise the act of suicide so that those who survived a suicide attempt would no longer be prosecuted. The man who led the change was Sir Charles Fletcher-Cooke who had been trying for over decade to decriminalise suicide, and the new law meant that those who attempted suicide could no longer be arrested though those who 'assisted, aided or abetted suicide' could be arrested and imprisoned for a term not exceeding fourteen years. Fletcher-Cooke, who had what would now be politely described as a colourful life (including at least one teenage boy), was a lawyer and politician who served as the constitutional adviser to Sultan Hassanal Bolkiah and went on to become a member of the European Parliament from 1977 to 1979 and a delegate to the European Council.

Since 1961, the law in England and Wales has been that although a patient is entitled to refuse treatment (even if that may lead to their death) active assistance in suicide is illegal. An individual cannot lawfully consent to anything more than the infliction of minor injury.

Suicide has gradually been decriminalised in other countries. It was, for example, decriminalised in Canada in 1972.

In the UK, there have been repeated attempts to make assisted suicide/euthanasia legal. The mainstream media seems to support euthanasia very strongly and opposing points of view do not seem to be aired very well.

As a result, there is a real chance that euthanasia will be legalised in the UK very soon. If and when that happens, doctors and nurses will make value judgements about the quality of other people's lives, while at the same time trying not to look as if they are tackling bed blocking, saving money and freeing up organs for transplantation.

And the DNR notices will still be used to free society of the people who are regarded as superfluous.

Numerous attempts have been made to legalise State controlled killing in the United Kingdom. One survey (conducted on behalf of a group campaigning for euthanasia) suggested that 90% of the public believed that euthanasia should be available. Such surveys will doubtless be used to support the campaign to introduce euthanasia into Britain.

However, ask different questions and use different words and I suspect that 90% of the public would oppose the legalisation of euthanasia.

Chapter Fifteen
Euthanasia in the USA

Euthanasia is alive and up and running in much of America. As in most countries it goes by many euphemisms.

They claim that in euthanasia the patient dies when the doctor gives a lethal injection but that in assisted suicide the doctor simply provides the lethal substance which the patient takes himself. Of course, if the patient's hand is shaking too much, the doctor will help by holding the patient's mouth open and pouring the poison down his or her throat. That still counts as assisted suicide.

In America, as elsewhere, death by doctor isn't being pushed by doctors but by politicians, lobbyists and lawyers. And they are using every trick in the book. Death by doctor is being sold as freedom, as a choice, as a human right. The people pushing for more euthanasia aren't people in pain. They are sometimes people who fear pain. But they are mostly people who have their own hidden reasons (usually financial) for promoting the idea.

Doctors themselves are mostly against the idea of the medical profession being involved. The American Medical Association and other major medical organisations have opposed the idea. Politicians are pushing hard, however, and are forcing doctors to accept euthanasia as a potential 'treatment' option.

It is said that the right to die in America has become the duty to die.

In Oregon and Washington, well over half of requests for assisted suicide cited 'feelings of being a burden' as significant reasons for their requests.

There can be absolutely no doubt that legally assisted suicide will lead to massive pressure on vulnerable, frightened individuals to accept the quick, cheap option of death over palliative care. And it must be remembered that where suicide has become legal, there has been a surge in the open solicitation of patients by those wanting their organs for someone else.

Just how enthusiastic would anyone be if doctors simply shot their patients in the head instead of injecting them?

A shot in the head would be more certain and probably less painful than the methods currently being used.

Or maybe gas chambers could be introduced. They are cheap and effective and proven and can be used to kill a number of people at a time.

Chapter Sixteen
Euthanasia is not painless, peaceful and dignified

It is a convenient myth (convenient for the proponents of euthanasia) that euthanasia (in its various forms and incarnations) is painless and dignified.

There is absolutely no evidence to show that it is either.

But there is plenty of evidence to show that it is neither.

Euthanasia does not provide the painless, peaceful death which its advocates claim it to be. There is no perfect way for the government to kill people. As Samuel Beckett said: 'Even death is unreliable'.

Here are 25 things everyone should know:

A study in the journal 'Anesthesia' reported that there were no standardised methods for euthanasia and so, as a result, there are frequent cases of prolonged and distressing deaths. There appears to be a high incidence of vomiting, re-awakening from coma and prolongation of the dying process (with some individuals taking up to seven days to die.)

In America, doctors cannot access drugs to use in cases of the death penalty because of cost and availability. International drug companies are unwilling to provide drugs intended to kill people on ethical grounds. (It is unusual to see drug companies citing 'ethical grounds' as a reason not to do something. I suspect that the real reason is that the drug companies are worried more about legal and reputational issues.)

Dr Bryan Betty, medical director of the Royal New Zealand College of GPs has warned that mixing concoctions of drugs has led to traumatic deaths.

There is considerable confusion about what to do if an initial attempt at euthanasia fails. Should the patient be told that they have to give their consent a second time? Or a third time? What should be done if a patient is semi-conscious and has not died? Should they then be kept alive? Or should another attempt be made to kill them?

A study performed in the Netherlands showed that in 21 of 114 cases, the patient did not die as soon as expected or woke up and the doctor had to kill them for a second time.

What happens if the doctor or nurse who is performing the euthanasia has left the building – which is likely to happen if a death takes a number of days?

What happens if a doctor or nurse cannot put an IV line into a vein? (This is something which often happens with elderly patients whose veins may be frail or damaged.)

The same drugs which are used for killing prisoners on death row are sometimes used to kill patients who have consented to euthanasia. But there is evidence that the killing of prisoners does not always go smoothly and can take longer than might be expected. (Lethal injections were introduced as more humane than the gas chamber or the electric chair. There is no evidence that they are.)

One of the drugs used in the authorised killing of patients is propofol which can sting as it flows through a vein when given in normal doses. No one knows what effect it has when given in large doses in euthanasia.

Dr Joel Zivot, an anesthesiologist and critical care doctor, has suggested that death by euthanasia could feel like drowning. If paralysing drugs are used, the patient appears calm, peaceful and quiet – but that doesn't tell us what the patient is experiencing.

When killing drugs are given orally, the death can take up to ten hours. If a doctor or nurse is not available with an IV kit ready, the distress to patients and relatives can be considerable.

People being killed by drugs may make gasping noises. 'We don't think they are signs of distress,' said Dr James Downar, a specialist in palliative and critical care. Note the word 'think'.

Monitors are not used when a patient is being killed. This means that there is no evidence about what is happening, and death can only be certified by a doctor or nurse feeling for a pulse. No attempts are made to monitor brain or cardiac response.

Autopsies of executed American prisoners show the accumulation of fluid in the lungs. This is very distressing, for the patient is effectively drowning in their own secretions.

Experts fear that patients being killed may suffer intolerable, unbearable physical or psychological pain.

In Belgium, the relatives of a 36-year-old woman heard screams when she was supposedly being euthanized. A post mortem showed that the woman had been suffocated with a pillow after the drugs failed to kill her.

An elderly, demented woman in Belgium was euthanized after her family decided that she should be killed. Since it was claimed that the woman didn't understand what was happening, the doctor laced her coffee with her sedatives – while she was chatting with her family. The doctor then gave another sedative by injection. The woman then stood up. Family members held her down while the doctor injected her and killed her. In court later the judges declared that 'given the deeply demented condition of the patient, the doctor did not need to verify her wish for euthanasia.' (I find it difficult to understand how this death could be described as euthanasia.)

A gunshot would be quicker and probably more painless than drugs. Why don't advocates of euthanasia endorse the idea that doctors should simply shoot patients? Patients could, like Nurse Edith Cavell, be put on a chair and shot in a scruffy courtyard. It would be faster and more certain than any other way of killing. A firing squad could be made up of doctors and nurses – with special fees for the occasion, of course.

In more than half of the cases where individuals in Oregon, USA were subjected to euthanasia, there is no record of whether or not there were any complications.

Complications which have been recorded during euthanasia include: difficulty in finding a vein, spasms, twitching, nausea, vomiting, tachycardia, sweating, gasping. One instance of euthanasia failed because the doctor had ordered the wrong drug. Another attempt was delayed when the doctor had to leave to fetch a second batch of lethal drugs.

Taking lethal drugs by mouth can be traumatic. It is not unusual for patients to take many hours to die. One patient took 104 hours to die. One patient became unconscious 25 minutes after swallowing lethal medication but woke up and regained consciousness 65 hours later.

One report showed that lethal injections caused severe pain and severe respiratory distress with associated sensations of drowning, asphyxiation, panic and terror in the overwhelming majority of cases. Dr Gail Van Norman has said that 'It is a virtual medical certainty that most, if not all, prisoners will experience excruciating suffering, including sensations of drowning and suffocation from pentobarbital.'

A study of more than 200 autopsy reports after executions in nine American States showed evidence of pulmonary oedema in the lungs (likely to cause a feeling of drowning or suffocation)

Midazolam used in executions has caused signs of pain – including gasping, choking and coughing, with patients heaving against their restraints.

Evidence shows that some people who choose assisted suicide vomit their lethal dose of drugs before it can be absorbed.

Chapter Seventeen
It's all about the money

The euthanasia scam is being sold as an exercise in kindness.

'The good news is that we can help you avoid pain and distress and save your family from the agony of seeing you decline slowly. By helping you to commit suicide, we bypass all that pain and take you straight to the closing credits.'

That's all nonsense, I'm afraid.

Euthanasia is all about money. It has been established that the average annual health care cost per person for individuals in their last year of life is 14 times as high as for those not in their last year of life.

As a result, money is being diverted from health care and palliative care into 'Voluntary Assisted Dying' programmes (also known as 'state sponsored deaths') which are designed to cut health care costs. It is a lot cheaper to kill people than it is to provide palliative care.

And, even more significantly, euthanasia programmes are being introduced in order to cut pension costs.

It is no secret that all developed countries are facing huge pension problems.

Many of those who receive State pensions believe (quite erroneously) that the money they have paid in taxes has been put aside to pay their pensions. In reality, of course, pension programmes are simply huge Ponzi schemes. The State pensions which are being paid today are paid out of today's taxes. And, in twenty years' time, the pensions which are paid out will be paid out of the taxes which are paid by workers in twenty years' time. If the size of the aged population can be cut, the annual savings will be measured in billions of dollars.

After thousands of elderly people were murdered in hospitals and care homes during the lockdowns, politicians boasted with glee that the financial savings, in unpaid pensions, would be huge. The more people they kill, the more money they'll save.

Let us all be honest about it: the pro-euthanasia programme is nothing to do with people's rights or with reducing pain or distress: it is, inevitably perhaps, all about money.

There are many ways in which the UK's National Health Service could save money. Sacking 20% of all the administrators would make no difference to the quality of care provided and would cut billions from the annual bill. Driving a harder bargain with drug companies would also save billions. And cutting waste would save billions too.

But none of these cost cutting schemes is as popular with bureaucrats as the introduction of legal euthanasia.

Rt Rev Iain Greenshields, moderator of the Church of Scotland has said that he is concerned that letting terminally ill patients legally end their lives would permanently change the NHS.

'Is this really the way we wish to see precious caring resource directed? Given the pressure on healthcare resources, we are also very concerned that assisted dying could be seen as providing an opportunity for cost saving.'

Rev Greenshields also said that passing a law approving of legally-assisted dying 'profoundly changes relationships not only between health professionals and patients, but also within families. We are concerned that, should assisted dying be legalised, the way our society views older people and those with disabilities will, over time, become more utilitarian.'

And the Rev Greenshields said that even with strict conditions in place, opening floodgates by passing any version of the law (to allow assisted dying) would likely result in later expansion.

The fear among many is that legally approved suicide would result in a massive increase in the number of people seeking assisted suicide due to poverty, homelessness or mental anguish. In Canada, more than a quarter of voters said that the poor and homeless should be allowed to end their lives with MAID. And there can be no doubt that legally assisted suicide would be used to solve immigrant and asylum seeker problems, and to deal with perceived over-crowding and over population problems.

It is naïve to assume that legally approved suicide would be restricted to helping the terminally, terminally ill to find a painless death.

Anyone who denies that all this is happening is either ignorant or hiding the truth in order to defend their enthusiasm for legally approved suicide.

'The take-away point is that there may be some upfront costs associated with offering medically assisted dying to Canadians, but there may also be a reduction in spending elsewhere in the system and therefore offering medical assistance in dying to Canadians will not cost the health care system anything extra,' said Aaron Trachtenberg, a resident in internal medicine and one of the authors of a report on assisted dying in Canada.

Astonishingly, a widely quoted Canadian report also stated that 'Hospital based care costs the health care system more than a comprehensive palliative care system where we could help people achieve their goal of dying at home.'

I found this astonishing for it seemed to assume that dying (whether by suicide or not) was an inevitable part of palliative care.

Everywhere in the world, administrators and doctors are drawing attention to the financial advantages that euthanasia can offer.

It is no secret that looking after the disabled, the frail and the elderly can be expensive. Politicians and the promoters of euthanasia claim that the provision of benefits, special buildings and staff mean that providing care has become a huge financial burden for national and local governments and for health care providers. The seriously disabled have to be provided with either comprehensive home care and support or with institutional care, usually in a purpose built building with many, highly trained (and therefore expensive) staff members. As populations have grown in size, so the number of people requiring care and the cost of providing that care has increased massively. And, of course, the seriously disabled individuals themselves are unlikely to be able to do anything to help themselves or to do productive work.

For many years now, the task of providing care for the disabled has been gradually but deliberately moved from governments onto voluntary groups. And yet the burden of the costs (often pushed higher by red tape, bureaucratic demands, minimum wages and so on) mean that facilities struggle to cope. Volunteers should be talking to patients, arranging flowers and generally making life better. Instead they are doing the cleaning and the washing up.

The provision of palliative care has suffered probably more than any other type of care, and administrators and doctors are now openly drawing attention to the real financial advantages which accrue if patients are persuaded to kill themselves (or, since many such patients may be physically incapable of killing themselves, to allow themselves to be killed).

None of this has come as a great surprise, of course.

Campaigners speaking on behalf of the disabled have for many decades warned that the legalisation of assisted suicide, and the extension of the legal boundaries, would lead to society devaluing the lives of people who are disabled (or frail, or elderly or anyone incapable of looking after themselves) and would make the disabled feel that they had a responsibility to kill themselves since their lives weren't worth living and they were taking up much needed resources. The usually unspoken fear was that patients would be made to feel guilty if they didn't kill themselves (or allow themselves to be killed).

And all this is now happening. And it is happening very rapidly.

Death is now seen as a viable alternative to costly and inevitably futile medical treatment.

A paper which appeared in the Canadian Medical Journal drew attention to this possibility very vividly. The authors concluded that Medically Assisted Death could reduce annual health spending by between $34.7 million and $136.8 million. (I always find it difficult to have any respect when such a wide range is offered. It suggests to me that the figures are no more than a guess.)

Moreover, it was pointed out that these savings would outweigh the estimated cost of implementing medically assisted dying by a considerable sum with the cost of offering euthanasia on a wide scale being estimated at between $1.5 million and $14.8 million. (Once again I had to check the figures since that seems to me to be a very wide range.)

Naturally, the authors of the report stressed that saving money should not be a consideration when considering whether a patient should live or die. But I am not the only observer to fear that this was merely an attempt to avoid official responsibility for the endless series of dilemmas which will now ensue and which will, I fear, be decided by people who are not unduly troubled by ethical niceties.

If the State wants a cull of the disabled, the incompetent, the frail, the elderly and the mentally ill then the State will have no difficulty in finding the people prepared to provide the cull.

Long waiting lists (getting longer in Canada as everywhere else), the effective rationing of medical services (with many operations only available for those who can pay privately) will mean that the pressure to execute euthanasia programmes on a wide scale will probably be well supported by the general public.

Suggesting that doctors and bureaucrats should not take financial problems into account is at best naïve and cynical. Doctors and bureaucrats already take cost into account, and it is now common for life-saving drugs to be unused simply because they cost too much.

The reality is that euthanasia is largely about saving money.

The slippery slope that campaigners have been warning about is very real. And we are already part of the way down the slope and we are moving faster down the slope each day.

The disabled and the elderly are now widely regarded as of little or no financial value.

Money has always had a much bigger effect on health and social care policies than is generally accepted. For example, in Britain, long stay residential homes for the mentally ill were closed because of political correctness. The result was that countless thousands of individuals who could not look after themselves were thrown out into the 'community'. A lack of services and help means that these unhappy souls now spend their days sitting in parks and bus shelters. They would spend their days in the public libraries except that there aren't many of those anymore. In reality, of course, this had nothing to do with political correctness. It was all about the money that could be saved.

The main reasons that people don't agree with the legalisation of euthanasia are a fear that vulnerable groups will be killed (or will be expected to put themselves forward in a Captain Oates sort of way to save money and resources) and a feeling that a doctor's role is to heal people and not to kill them. (Captain Lawrence Oates was the Antarctic Explorer who in 1912, when suffering from frostbite and gangrene, walked out into the snow, leaving his three companions in their tent in the hope that by doing so he would increase their chances of survival. He chose death rather than the prospect of being a burden on his companions. As he left the tent Oates said: 'I am going outside and may be some time.' It was his birthday.)

Independent studies and surveys have repeatedly shown that less than 10% of people support legalisation, and when they do they do so largely because they are wrongly convinced that euthanasia can prevent inevitable and unavoidable pain and suffering during terminal illnesses.

Finally, there is one other reason why the establishment is so keen on euthanasia: it will release a good many organs for use.

Two controversial researchers (Dr David Shaw an ethicist at the Universities of Basel and Maastricht and Professor Alec Morton, a health economist) have argued that killing terminally ill patients would release organs for transplantation – as well as saving money. They argue that changing the legislation to allow more assisted suicide would benefit the people who want to die and the larger general population.

The two authors wrote: 'Organ donation could also benefit because there are several reasons why donation, after assisted dying, is better from a clinical and economic perspective. First, if patients are denied assisted dying, organ function will gradually deteriorate until they died naturally, meaning that transplantation is less likely to be successful. Second, patients who choose assisted dying have to go through a lengthy process and organ donation can be easily integrated into that process.'

It has been revealed in Canada that the legalisation of assisted suicide has led to the open solicitation of those considering medically assisted death. In one instance, a chronically ill man was denied health care at home and offered an assisted suicide. There is no little irony in the fact that patients being encouraged to die might themselves be saved if they were considered important enough to be treated as organ recipients rather than as organ donors.

Dr Moira McQueen, executive director of the Canadian Catholic Bioethics Institute said that a primary physician 'might well suggest organ donation as, if not an incentive, kind of 'consolation' for the person's own loss of life.'

Since organ transplantation is extremely expensive, and health services are cutting costs, it is inevitable that the organs taken from patients who have been murdered by the State will be reserved for politicians, bureaucrats and others who are regarded as, and treated as, important individuals.

Please excuse my cynicism. I have been practising medicine for a long time and I know how the system works.

Chapter Eighteen
Who will be allowed to kill themselves?

In New Zealand, patients who opt for euthanasia 'must be over 18 years of age, have a terminal illness which is likely to end their life within six months, be experiencing unbearable suffering and have the capacity to make an informed decision'.

Officially, doctors are supposed to encourage patients to talk to their family about the decision but under the law they do not have to discuss their intentions with anyone.

The flaws in all this are obvious to anyone with medical experience.

First, no doctor can say with certainty that a patient will die within six months. When I was a GP I had two patients who were told that they had just months to live but who were alive many years later. In both cases investigations suggested that the patients concerned were unlikely to live long. (In one instance, I had a phone call from the laboratory asking me why I had sent them a blood sample from a patient who was dead. I then gave up sending more blood samples for testing. The patient was still alive many years later when I retired from general practice.)

Second, the whole purpose of palliative care is to treat suffering and pain, and experts are very good at doing this, while allowing the patient to remain alert and reasonably active.

Third, it is difficult to know whether anyone can make an informed decision to kill themselves.

There are many aspects to the euthanasia programmes which I find scary but one of the scariest is, perhaps, the notion that lives can now be ended if a health professional considers that the individual's life is pointless. They call this 'the completed life' syndrome. The idea is that although the individual may be physically and mentally healthy, they feel disappointed with their lives. They feel that they have not achieved much, that their expectations have not been met and that they would have liked a better life.

Many of those who are described as 'tired of life' have lost hope and are in fear of being a burden. They consider themselves a burden, unwanted and unloved.

And instead of encouraging them to look for ways in which they might be able to enrich their lives, society offers them death as an easy, over-in-a-moment, solution that costs very little and is cheaper than any other answer.

Those who promote the idea of euthanasia claim that it is being offered as a compassionate solution for all the problems which doctors and society cannot solve. (There is no little irony in the fact that in the 1970s and 1980s in particular, benzodiazepine tranquillisers were prescribed by the ton as a solution to all the problems for which doctors could not offer solutions. Today, benzodiazepines are part of the killing solution for benzodiazepine drugs such as midazolam are often offered as part of the killing regime.)

It is worth noting too, that when a doctor refuses to help a patient kill themselves, that patient will be free to attend one of the many private clinics which have opened up and which offer euthanasia in much the same way that other private clinics offer breast enlargements or liposuction. These clinics claim to be offering 'the ultimate help'.

And if that doesn't alarm you, consider this.

As I have mentioned before in this book, the enthusiasts are even killing children.

Doctors from Toronto have outlined policies and procedures for 'medically assisted death for children.

Back in 2018, the British Medical Journals 'Journal of Medical Ethics' published an article in which doctors from Toronto's Hospital for Sick Children described plans to administer medically assisted death to children. They even described situations where the parents would not be informed until after the child had died.

The paper appeared before the Canadian Council of Academies was preparing to report to the Canadian Parliament about extending voluntary euthanasia or assisted dying to patients under the age of 18 (otherwise widely known as children), to psychiatric patients (patients who are mentally ill and generally considered to be unable to make important decisions) and patients who had expressed a preference for euthanasia but who had been rendered incapable of making the decision because of dementia or some other disease.

Written by paediatricians, administrators (!) and ethicists (!) the paper does not concern itself with discussion with parents before death – leaving this to the 'reflection period' after the child or mentally ill patient has been legally killed.

Bizarrely, the argument against asking parents for their help in making a decision is the old chestnut of patient confidentiality. The authors of the paper say that if a child doesn't want its parents involved then their wishes must be respected.

The authors of the paper argue that since Ontario does not require parents to be involved if a child decides they don't want further treatment then there is no legal reason to require parental involvement if the child has decided to die.

The cruel absurdity of this program of paediatric genocide or assassination is heightened by the universal knowledge that there cannot have ever been a child who has not, at one point or another thought or said: 'I wish I were dead'. Children who are in pain (with a stomach ache or toothache), children who are worried about examinations and teenagers whose hormones are turning them inside out are all likely to feel this way. And these days, children are made to worry more than ever.

Chapter Nineteen
Who will do the Killing?

Since all good doctors and nurses refuse to have anything to do with euthanasia, who is going to do the actual killing?

I suspect that many of the people who will be attracted to this bizarre and counter-intuitive branch of medicine will be psychopaths.

In the same way that both the army and the police force are known to attract a certain number of psychopathic individuals who are attracted by the idea of being able to kill people quite legally, there is no doubt that euthanasia programmes will attract would-be murderers, assassins and killers. There will be a new medical speciality, comprised almost exclusively of doctors and nurses who, like the notorious Dr Harold Shipman (the British general practitioner who killed hundreds of his patients before being exposed) will enjoy killing people.

And just what precautions will be in place to ensure that this new, small army of peripatetic psychopaths do not encourage their victims to give them items of value or to change their wills in their favour?

Who is going to be trained to help with euthanasia?

In New Zealand, after a referendum showed 65% support for the End of Life Choice Act, a survey organised by the Ministry of Health and which involved nearly 2,000 health care practitioners, showed that fewer than one third of health care practitioners were prepared to participate in the proposed 'assisted dying' regime. (Theoretically, any registered doctor or nurse will count as a 'medical practitioner' who is able to kill patients or help them kill themselves.)

The problem, of course, is that good, caring doctors and nurses are trained to keep people alive and not to kill them and any genuine, honest health care professional has to have grave doubts about the intentions and level of dedication of anyone prepared to spend their days helping patients die instead of helping to keep them alive. In reality, experts believe that the number of doctors prepared to help patients to die will be considerably less than a third of the total. Moreover, 33 of New Zealand's hospices were refusing to have anything to do with euthanasia. Some clinicians have said that they would rather leave medicine than be involved in any way with euthanasia.

Palliative care specialists agree that most of those who are skilled in end of life care want nothing to do with euthanasia. Dr Catherine D'Souza, of the Australian and New Zealand Society of Palliative Medicine, warns that this will leave patients in the hands of people who are not experts in end of life care or of pain management.

The result of this shortage is that euthanasia is going to be unavailable in some areas of the country. And because that will not be acceptable to politicians, one of two things will happen. Or both will happen.

First, euthanasia will be provided by a small group of itinerant doctors who will travel around the country killing patients. These doctors will know nothing about the patients they see. They will be the modern equivalent of the professional hangmen who used to travel around with a supply of rope and a complete absence of compassion.

Second, euthanasia will be provided by specialists who, it is claimed, will have as little as six hours' online training. And this will, without doubt, result in patients ending their lives because they are in pain when they have not had a chance to speak with a palliative care specialist who is able to control their pain. The euthanasia specialists who are not qualified doctors will not, of course, be legally allowed to prescribe suitable life-ending drugs.

It seems likely that New Zealand, and other countries which allow patients to make the decision to kill themselves will, as has happened in Australia, require that those intending to offer euthanasia take only a brief course. In Victoria, Australia, potential euthanasia specialists need only take an online six hour training course.

So, the bottom line is that euthanasia will, when offered by suitably qualified specialists, be available only in certain areas of any country. In other areas there may be no euthanasia service or it will be provided by people who are itinerant, professional killers with little or no knowledge of palliative care or of the needs and rights of patients and relatives.

Chapter Twenty
Palliative care is a basic human right

Palliative care is a basic human right and it is (or should be) an obligation of all governments to provide access to necessary health care facilities and services.

According to the United Nations Special Rapporteur on Torture, denying access to suitable and necessary pain relief can amount to inhuman and degrading treatment which is akin to torture.

Palliative care is needed for long-term patients as well as for patients with life-limiting and life-threatening illnesses, and there should be no time or prognostic limit on the delivery of palliative care. Most importantly, palliative care should be integrated with treatment programmes and curative care.

It has been estimated that in any one year, the number of patients requiring palliative care is around 40 million. There are, however, only around 13,000 palliative care organisations in the world (including hospices) and these manage to provide care for considerably less than 10% of the 40 million.

Moreover, the number of available palliative care beds and professionals is shrinking rather than growing as money is moved away from palliative care and into suicide programmes and the recruitment and paying of professional assassins to help with the killing when patients find it difficult to kill themselves.

Most palliative care is, of course, provided in North America, Europe and Australasia. It is estimated that 75% of countries have no or completely inadequate access to strong analgesics. Without oral opioids, effective palliative care is virtually impossible.

(The controversy surrounding the over-prescribing of oral opioids, particularly in the USA, has meant that more and more doctors are unwilling to prescribe oral opioids even to patients who have significant pain. The excuse is that prescribing strong painkillers can lead to addiction and the easiest way to avoid this problem is not to prescribe strong painkillers at all. The result is that people who are in severe pain and who are not given pain relief will accept euthanasia.)

There is a clear plan in the UK to reduce the amount of palliative care available in order to push patients into accepting euthanasia – even when they could enjoy many months or even years of productive, enjoyable life.

The euthanasia plan is part of the depopulation plan and anyone suggesting otherwise is naïve.

The evidence for this claim is widespread and growing.

For example, hospices across the north west of England are facing a funding crisis with 29 of the 30 hospices in the region warning of a budget shortfall. They say that vital services will need to be cut unless more funding is forthcoming. However, the Department of Health and Social Care says it is up to local health care boards to decide how much money goes into end-of-life care.

Government funding for adult hospice services has fallen by £47 million in the last two years while at the same time the number of people requiring hospice care is increasing. One hospital alone, says that they need to raise around £12,000 a week (more than £4 million a year) to stay open. And that money is raised from volunteers selling flags, shaking collecting tins and selling donated items. In the UK, the NHS used to provide £1 for every £2 raised by a hospice but gradually the contribution from the NHS has fallen. Today, the NHS, which is awash with money and which pays huge armies of pen-pushing administrators vast salaries in excess of £100,000 a year, contributes less than 70 pence for every £2 raised by volunteers. The money raised isn't used for luxuries – it is needed for medicines, for equipment, for food and for utilities. 'A new cupboard for controlled drugs cost about five to six thousand pounds,' said a doctor running one hospice. 'We have to raise that money ourselves.'

'It is absurd,' said one doctor, 'that hospices should have to find three quarters of their funding themselves. Just imagine the outcry if, for example, maternity services relied on jumble sales, car boot sales, bucket collections and charity shops to survive. Why should hospice services be treated as an added extra in the health service, rather than as the essential service they assuredly are?

Even MPs realise that the situation for hospices is unrealistic and close to impossible. The UK's All Party Parliamentary Group for Hospice and End of Life Care published a report in January 2024 which concluded that the current funding model for hospices was not fit for purpose and that, consequently, the services they provide are at risk. The Parliamentary Group concluded that 'the UK Government must provide a national plan to ensure the right funding flows to hospices'.

But, almost inevitably and certainly predictably, nothing has happened and hospices are having to close some of their beds. The result of that is that patients have to use NHS hospital beds. And many of those patients will be under tremendous pressure to accept 'end of life care' – which is a synonym for death.

Data collected from Integrated Care Boards across England shows that hospice funding has fallen in real terms in every part of the country in the last two years. ICBs have a statutory obligation to provide funding for palliative and end of life care appropriate to the local needs.

They have, however, failed in this.

Hospices provide care and support and essential nursing for 300,000 people a year in the UK. But those hospices remain largely funded by charity. Not one ICB has provided an increase in the money provided to hospices which matches inflation. Some ICBs have offered no increase at all.

It is quite clear that the aim is to reduce palliative care just as the availability of euthanasia is increased.

By May 2023, some of New Zealand's biggest hospices were warning that they would have to cut services if they didn't receive money from the Government.

There were reported to be between seven and nine full-time equivalent members of staff dedicated to euthanasia and two palliative care full-time equivalent members of staff for the 30,000 patients who were dying and need palliative care.

Things are so bad that one big hospice for years had buckets to catch water dripping from holes in the roof. Only when a former resident died and left a chunk of money could the roof be repaired.

In NZ as in the UK, hospices have to find most of the money they need themselves and so they are cutting back. They only take patients at the end of their lives because they cannot afford to look after them for many months, and they can't provide bereavement counselling for relatives.

In March 2023, it was announced that hospices in the UK would spend almost £200 million more on delivering care than they would receive in income. Nearly every hospice in the UK was said to be spending more than it was receiving. The shortfall is in a great part due to the failure of the Government to keep hospices properly funded. (The NHS only provides around a third of the money needed to run hospices but the NHS is no longer providing the money it should. Insufficient NHS support will inevitably mean that hospices will close or have to reduce the services they provide.)

Just imagine the furore if clinics providing infertility services, advice for diabetics, or cosmetic surgery were only able to function if they received money raised from bring-and-buy sales, jumble sales and street collections.

Hospices shouldn't just be a place to die. They should be a place where people who are seriously ill and perhaps don't have long to live can be in peace, without pain and enjoy a good quality of life. And although hospices mostly deal with residential patients, some also provide services for patients who come in once or twice a week to talk and be with other people.

But, I repeat, hospices rely on volunteers to raise money, run shops, drive patients to appointments, serve meals, record life stories, coordinate with relatives.

Hospitals are terrible places for people who are ill and either recovering or for whom no other treatment is available.

There is one other serious problem.

In some areas, it is clear that hospices which refuse to use professional assassins to kill their patients will lose their funding.

In Canada, a hospice had its funding withdrawn after it refused to offer euthanasia and assisted suicide to its patients.

Health authorities in Canada are saving huge amounts of money by killing patients and are putting money saving above the freedom of patients to die free from the threat of assassination.

Hospices in Canada, like the UK and most of the rest of the world, rely on donations and volunteers. And, of course, hospices relieve pressure on hospital beds

Hospitals are expensive because they have hugely expensive equipment, operating theatres and numerous skilled and expensive technicians, plus whole armies of incredibly expensive bureaucrats (whose role sometimes seem to consist of making life difficult for doctors and uncomfortable for patients). And it is in hospitals, rather than hospices, that patients are mostly at risk of being killed.

As you might by now expect, palliative care funding is being cut in Australia too.

In Australia the NSW Government is cutting its budget for end of life care by $150 million. One district in Sydney is having its palliative care funding cut by 30%.

The news about palliative care funding appeared in October 2023, during a debate about the introduction of the mass, legalised slaughter of the elderly and the sick. (Actually, the debate was officially about the introduction of 'voluntary assisted dying'. But since politicians and modern journalists use spin on a daily basis, it seems reasonable for me to tell the truth in a blunt fashion.)

A retired palliative care physician Dr Philip Lee said 'there was depression among local health services at the decision to cut the extra funding'. He said it would mean plans to recruit extra palliative staff would have to be paused and appointments cancelled.'

Dr Lee queries whether it would lead to more referrals to 'voluntary assisted dying' because there would be more patients whose palliative care needs are not met.

(It is interesting to note that most of the doctors who are speaking out about the reduction in facilities for palliative care are, like the doctors who are speaking out against 'voluntary assisted dying' and the doctors who spoke out against the covid lockdowns, the unscientific use of masks and the mass distribution of an inadequately tested vaccine, have been in practice for some years. They are the only doctors with the courage to stand up and tell the truth.)

Every health professional should understand the requirements, the theory and the practice of palliative care. But palliative care is still not widely taught in medical schools and nursing schools, and social workers, religious workers and psychologists are taught little or nothing about this vital aspect of care. Moreover, palliative care is almost exclusively controlled not by governments (which have the statutory responsibility to provide proper care for their citizens) but by private sector health care and by charities. (In contrast, medical schools are teaching would-be doctors about how to practise euthanasia.)

Ideally, palliative care should be an integral part of all primary care. It should be essential, compulsory and widely available and not regarded as an optional extra. Almost all pain, including severe pain, can be treated if the facilities and the will are there. But they are not.

The primary problem in many countries is that family doctor services have become available for the sort of hours that accountancy services are available.

In the UK, for example, GPs now work for an average of 25 hours a week. Very few doctors provide any care at night, at weekends or on bank holidays.

If care is available for just 25 hours a week, this inevitably means that for 143 hours a week, patients who are in pain have no access to palliative care or, indeed, any kind of medical care.

All around the world the figures are the same and show that most people would like to die at home. Traditionally, most people did die at home, surrounded by the things they've lived with and loved and, most importantly, with their loved ones beside them. However, what happens is exactly the opposite – most people die in hospitals or nursing homes and a few die in hospices or palliative care homes.

Those who would prefer to die at home should look at buying necessary equipment (a hospital bed, a hoist and so on) with the money which would be spent on buying nursing home care. Grants may be available in some areas.

What the world desperately needs, of course, is more mobile palliative care services with doctors and nurses available to visit patients who are dying and who are in their own homes. Even if elderly patients are not living alone (and many are) their spouses are likely to be elderly and frail and unable to provide all the necessary care without help.

But exactly the opposite is happening.

And nowhere illustrates this more vividly than Britain.

Just a few decades ago, general practitioners used to be available to visit their patients at home during the daytime, during the evening, at weekends and on bank holidays. Nowhere in the world was there a better 24 hour a day GP service than in Britain. The GP service was, indeed, widely recognised to be the very best part of the National Health Service. The family doctor (a concept now, sadly, simply a memory) would be available to visit, to provide advice and to send in a nurse whenever this seemed appropriate and necessary. If the family doctor was off duty one of his partners (who would, at the very least, have access to the patient's notes) would visit.

All that changed dramatically when general practitioners were given the opportunity to stop visiting patients at home and decided to stop providing out of hours service. (Things are actually worse than that. Many doctors in Britain, terrified of catching a disease from a patient, refuse to see patients at all and insist on providing only a telephone service. This, of course, is an entirely inadequate substitute, and although some young doctors fail to understand this, it is impossible for a doctor to make a reliable diagnosis over the telephone.)

Even those doctors who are willing to see patients in their surgery or clinic, work very abbreviated hours and today, the average GP earns well over £100,000 a year and, as I have already explained, works just 24 or 25 hours a week.

Many patients have found that the only contact they ever have with their GP is when she or he contacts them to arrange an appointment with a nurse to have one of the many, exceedingly profitable, vaccinations which are now a regular £50,000 to £100,000 bonus for GPs (even though they don't do any of the vaccinating themselves).

Allowing family doctors to stop doing what family doctors have always done has destroyed health care in Britain. It has meant that there is more untreated illness, that more people are suffering from chronic illnesses, and that more are suffering unnecessarily and are dying of treatable disorders. It is destruction of the GP service which has led directly to the destruction of the ambulance service and the hospital service – with the result that in Britain today there is, effectively, no functioning health care. The refusal of GPs to provide a proper 24 hour a day service means that patients have little alternative but to call for an ambulance or visit their nearest Accident and Emergency hospital department. Many of these patients have problems which could be dealt with by a GP in five minutes but the vastly increased pressure on these services means that the average waiting time for an ambulance has gone in many areas from minutes to hours, and the average waiting time in Accident and Emergency departments is now ten, eleven, twelve or more hours with a growing number of patients waiting days to be seen. It is now by no means exceptional for patients to die in

Accident and Emergency departments while waiting to be treated. All these problems are a direct result of the decision by GPs to stop providing the out-of-hours service that was previously required in their terms of service.

And, again, as I have already implied, the problem for the elderly and the very sick is that doctors are reluctant to prescribe painkillers such as opioids because of the publicity which has been given to the opioid addiction problem. The fact is that drug addiction is never a problem when drugs are being prescribed for patients in severe pain and when patients are terminally ill there is clearly no problem.

And the end result of all this is a dramatic increase in the number of patients who are left in pain, distress and despair. It is no secret, and no surprise, that Britain now has the worst record in the world for treating cancer patients. It is now no longer unusual for patients with stage four cancer to have to wait six months before they receive any treatment – if they are still alive. And that appalling service (or lack of service) within the State health service has led, inevitably, to an increase in the number of patients who are asking to be allowed to die. Of course, politicians, celebrities and members of the royal family do not have to wait six months for treatment. They can safely expect that their treatment will start within hours if not minutes of a diagnosis being made.

The dramatic deterioration of the GP service has destroyed health care in Britain.

The destruction of health services provided in Britain is not unique. The same deterioration has taken place around the world and it has led to a dramatic increase in the number of people agreeing to have Do Not Resuscitate notices placed on their medical records and accepting euthanasia as the only viable option.

I was a GP for many years in a small practice and I considered myself privileged. I was constantly rewarded by my relationship with my patients whom I considered to be members of my extended family. I know that my professional colleagues felt the same way. I now feel betrayed by the new generation of GPs who have chosen to abandon the traditional role of the family doctor, and it is a cause of great sadness to me that they feel no sense of vocation and that their dedication appears to be their bank balances rather than to their patients. It is not surprising that the majority of patients no longer trust or respect their doctors. I also feel sorry for the doctors who have abandoned the responsibilities which it is their duty to accept. They have lost the joy of being in general practice, for the joy came from the relationship which a doctor can traditionally enjoy with his patients. My happiest moments as a GP came after visiting patients at home, at a weekend or at night, and being able to make a difference. I doubt if young doctors ever know the feeling of making a difference. That is their great loss.

Patients lost a great deal when doctors decided to abandon their traditional role. But I suspect that doctors lost even more.

Today, the only hope for at-home palliative care comes from charities and mobile hospice services which can send nurses and other care staff into the homes of those who need support. The medical profession has abandoned those it was created to serve.

And if you doubt that the hidden agenda of those supporting the euthanasia movement is simply to kill as many people as possible, to reduce the global population and to get rid of the elderly, the disabled, the frail, the dependent and the expensive, consider this: It would cost no more than the cost of a couple of nights' stay in a hospital to provide patients at home with hospital beds, hoists and all the other equipment needed to nurse them in their own surroundings efficiently and lovingly. And it would cost no more than the cost of a couple more nights' stay in a hospital, or the cost of a couple of overpaid bureaucrats, to provide a team of community nurses able to visit patients at home.

But that will never happen because it doesn't fit the plan.

Oh, and one other thing.

Professor Rod MacLeod, a Palliative Care specialist, who has been in practice for over 30 years has said that nearly every week that he has spent working in hospice care he has been approached by someone who wanted to end their life but all but one of those individuals later changed their minds when they were offered and provided with proper palliative care. Professor MacLeod says that when euthanasia is widely available, people will be put to death who would have changed their minds.

Chapter Twenty One
Basic truths about euthanasia

1) By an astonishing coincidence, and just as happened with the covid fraud, exactly the same things are happening all around the world. Euthanasia is being promoted and legalised all around the world (just as the covid fraud was promoted globally)
2) The media is promoting a superficial, one-sided view of euthanasia as a way to relieve pain and distress.
3) Palliative care, offered to patients who are seriously or terminally ill, is being defunded.
4) The number of patients developing cancer (and requiring care) has increased dramatically. The use of masks, and the resultant hypoxia, resulted in cancers being more dangerous than ever. Many newly diagnosed patients are suffering from fast growing cancers. There can now be no doubt that many cases of cancer are caused by the covid-19 'vaccine'. As the number of patients increases, so the quality of care provided decreases.
5) The covid fraud led to an increase in compliance – with the majority of people now prepared to do whatever they are told to do ('have a vaccine', 'wear a mask', 'stay at home', etc.). The people who were compliant during the pandemic will be compliant when offered euthanasia.
6) The official incidence of mental illness is increasing very rapidly – particularly among children and young people. Laws concerning euthanasia are being changed so that the mentally ill can be accepted as candidates for death.
7) Laws concerning euthanasia are being changed so that children can decide to kill themselves without their parents' knowledge or ability to intervene.
8) Politicians and doctors' trade unions have deliberately and systematically destroyed primary care. And as a result, other health services everywhere have failed the public with the quality and quantity of services having deteriorated

Chapter Twenty Two
Why euthanasia should be illegal and why you should oppose it

1) There is no known way of killing people in a peaceful, painful and dignified way.
2) In whichever country a law is passed legalising euthanasia, the parameters are likely to be extended quite soon afterwards. So, for example, if a law is passed legalising the killing of patients at the very end of their lives, the law will be extended to cover patients who are not terminally ill. And then the law will be extended to cover the mentally ill and to include children.
3) There is evidence that patients who are not ready to die will be bullied into accepting euthanasia.
4) The poor and those requiring benefit payments and State support will probably be bullied or blackmailed into accepting euthanasia.
5) Relatives who want to benefit from an elderly person's estate will arrange euthanasia for mercenary reasons.
6) Hospitals which want to free up beds will feel free to kill patients.
7) There is a risk, too, that people who arrive at a hospital in an ambulance, having been given a powerful painkiller or tranquilliser, will be invited straightaway to accept a doctor-assisted suicide. And, because they are confused and frightened, they will accept the offer without properly understanding the consequences. Doctors involved in patient care should never, ever be involved in promoting, selling or even discussing euthanasia.
8) Some advocates of euthanasia claim that candidates for suicide must have a fatal illness. And some euthanasia programmes begin by saying that a patient must be expected to be dead within six months. Campaigners say that this excludes patients who might live for years. They're wrong, of course. They're wrong because prognoses are subjective and they are wrong more often than they are right. I could fill London with people who have been told to prepare themselves for death but who have lived for many years. The

advocates for euthanasia assume that it is possible to decide that an illness is fatal. Anyone (doctor or nurse) who announces that an illness is fatal is a fool. I doubt if I am alone in having seen patients who have been told that they were incurable, recover and enjoy long lives – not uncommonly outliving the physician who had told them they were dying. Diagnostic errors are nowhere near as rare as doctors would like to imagine. Dr Vernon Coleman has described how he was wrongly diagnosed with kidney cancer and given six months to live. That was nearly 40 years ago. In fact the radiologists who had made the diagnosis were wrong. Politicians seem to assume that it is possible to predict when a patient is going to die. It isn't. Very occasionally, a patient will conveniently die as predicted but this, I suspect, is more due to the voodoo or negative placebo factor than due to any brilliance on the part of the forecaster. Doctors, like witch doctors, can have a powerful influence on the outcome of an illness if they give a patient a firm and professional sounding prognosis. In other words, if a doctor says to a patient: 'You will be dead in six months' there is a chance that the patient will be dead in six months because the doctor said so. It is rare for patients to die before a forecasting doctor suggests but it is common for patients to live considerably longer. Selecting a patient as suitable for euthanasia on the basis of a prognosis is always dangerous and unjustifiable. Examples of mistaken diagnoses and erroneous prognoses are not difficult to find. A 45-year-old mother of two was told that she had an inoperable tumour on her liver. With no family present she was told that she had between two months and two years to live. (How any doctor can offer such a bizarrely wide prognosis is difficult to understand.) In fact she had a benign liver tumour. She was not told of the error for a month. It was a year before the woman had recovered from the trauma of the mistaken diagnosis. But what if she had been persuaded to accept euthanasia? Another woman who was told that she had terminal cancer was found to be suffering from sarcoidosis. Once again a wrong diagnosis had been made and this time the patient was treated with toxic chemotherapy and subjected to frequent CT scans and medical reviews. The mistaken diagnosis was maintained for four years. A third woman who had a history of breast cancer was told that the cancer had returned and had spread to her lungs. She underwent treatment, including radiotherapy. After five years of believing that she could die at any moment, the woman was told that the hospital had made a mistake and that she actually had bronchiectasis. A 51-year-old man was told that he had advanced amyotrophic lateral sclerosis (ALS). A second doctor agreed with the diagnosis which had been made on the basis of a 10 minute examination. The man was told that he would never return to work and would soon be unable to walk. He was contacted by a therapist regarding medically assisted death and began to plan music for his funeral. The man closed his business and told his friends and family the terrible news. He was told that he would not live until the following Christmas. Eventually the man saw a third doctor who told him that he had been misdiagnosed and actually had neuropathy caused by his diabetes. A 65-year-old man was diagnosed with Motor Neurone Disease and told that he was terminally ill with just six months to live. He was told to choose a hospice. He later found that his symptoms were actually caused by the statins he was taking. When he'd been told he was terminally ill he stopped the statins and his symptoms disappeared. These case histories are by no means unusual. In countries where assisted killing is in place there will, without doubt, be instances where misdiagnosed patients will choose euthanasia and will die quite unnecessarily. One of the main objections to capital punishment (a process which often takes many years and repeated examinations of the evidence) is the fear that a mistake will be made and an innocent person will be killed. The same objection can and should be raised about medically assisted dying.

Finally, to summarise, you should oppose euthanasia if:
You are over 60 years of age or hope or expect to be over 60 years of age one day
You ever feel glum or down in the dumps, upset, worried, fearful or tired of life
You are forgetful or absent minded
You have any health problem (diabetes, arthritis, breathing troubles, heart problems, poor vision, poor hearing or incontinence to name but a small selection)
All of those problems and situations could enable doctors and nurses to kill you for your 'own comfort' and to do so without asking your permission.

You can make a difference and help stop the horror of doctor-assisted suicide by sharing the truth. Make sure everyone you know reads this book to understand what is happening to us all.

Appendix: The Author

'Jack King' is the nom de plume of a former British GP principal who was a doctor for over 40 years and who is now retired. Anyone who questions the establishment is likely to find themselves struck off the medical register (as it used to be called) or to have their licence taken away (as it is now known). Jack King writes: 'Instead of protecting patients and the reputation of the medical profession, the GMC now seems to me to exist to protect the pharmaceutical industry and the British Government. I want to be able to work as a locum occasionally and to continue giving advice whenever and wherever I can. I have therefore, reluctantly, adopted a nom de plume, to protect my identity and to provide myself with protection against the authorities in general but particularly against the GMC. My identity has been well hidden.'

The name Dr Cicely Marsden is also a nom de plume of a British doctor.

Printed in Great Britain
by Amazon